Skiing the North Shore

A guide to cross-country trails in Minnesota's
spectacular Lake Superior region

SECOND EDITION

ANDREW SLADE

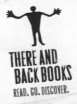

**THERE AND
BACK BOOKS**
READ. GO. DISCOVER.

Duluth, Minnesota

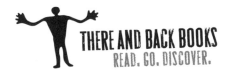

There & Back Books, Duluth, Minnesota
bestnorthshore.com

This book is dedicated to the trail groomers —
they brave the dawn, fix the snow machines,
and work for love or peanuts
so that we all can enjoy these trails.

Contents

NORTH SHORE MOUNTAINS: Everything is Connected

GUNFLINT TRAIL: Ski-In Hospitality

Foreword

I remember the day vividly. Crystal blue. Perfect tracks. Temperature in the upper 20s.

Half a dozen of us were rocking and rolling along the intimate Korkki Nordic ski trails between Duluth and Superior. We were classic skiing—the only kind of skiing you can do on these trails among the balsam fir and aging aspen.

The sun was making diamonds on the snow. The kick was good. The glide was better. I think all of us knew it might be the best day of skiing we would have all winter. Certainly, it would have been hard to top it.

I have no doubt that skiers all along the North Shore were having similar experiences on other trails. Up at the Erkki Harju Trail in Two Harbors. Along the North Shore Mountains Trails. Up at Pincushion on the hill above Grand Marais.

We are fortunate, here on the North Shore of Lake Superior, to have an amazing variety of cross-country ski trails and, in most winters, plenty of snow to complement them. Most of us have our "home" trails, the ones that we can get to quickly for a spin before dark, or even a lighted loop that we can do after work.

But every now and then, we want to discover new country and different tracks. That's why this book by Andrew Slade is just what we need. We can keep it handy on the shelf at home or throw it in the daypack when we want to forge into new territory.

The maps and trail descriptions let us know exactly what we're getting into. Are the trails easy or difficult? Which loops are okay for the kids? What kind of views and scenery can we expect? How's the grooming likely to be? Is there a lodge or restaurant nearby?

Those are the questions we have when we venture onto new trails, and this book answers them.

But perhaps equally important, just looking at all of the trails waiting for us, we'll be inspired to get out and enjoy North Shore skiing even more than we already do.

Sam Cook — Duluth, Minnesota

Introduction

Minnesota's North Shore of Lake Superior is home to some of the best cross-country skiing in North America. A billion years ago, a lucky bit of geology created the rugged topography of the Sawtooth Mountains. The glaciers of the last Ice Age created the world's largest freshwater lake, Lake Superior. Eventually, Scandinavian immigrant families arrived here to log the land and fish the waters—and they built Nordic ski trails like nowhere else.

Today, with abundant snowfall from moisture off of Lake Superior, and with over seven hundred kilometers of perfectly groomed ski trails near the shore, you'll find a world-class skiing experience that won't disappoint.

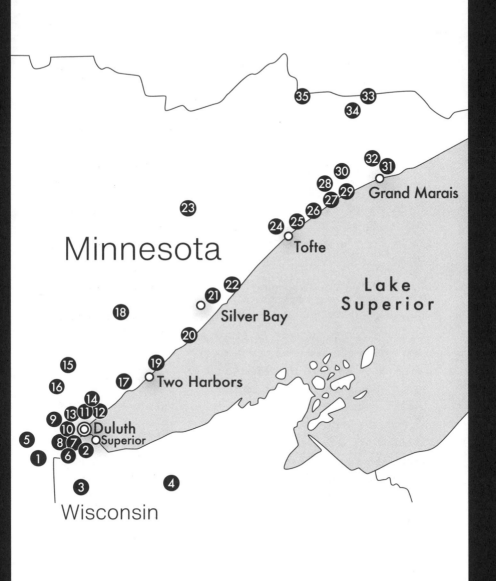

Why is North Shore skiing so darn good? Why do intelligent people give up on career advancement just to live near these trails? Why do families drive five hours each way for a few glorious hours in these woods?

There's no single answer to these questions. It's the rugged scenery and remote terrain. It's the winter weather, bringing more reliable snowfall to the North Shore than anywhere else in the state. It's the traditional hospitality passed down from generations.

A massive geologic event over one billion years ago created the foundation of the North Shore's current landscape. Layer after layer of lava and magma erupted from a huge rift in the earth's crust. These layers stacked up 20,000 feet high, then tilted in toward the center of what is now Lake Superior.

Glaciers from the last Ice Age scoured these layers down, leaving distinct ridges and valleys known now as the Sawtooth Mountains. The glaciers left behind the basin for the world's largest expanse of fresh water, Lake Superior.

The broad inland sea that settled next to these rugged ridges created the perfect combination of dramatic views and lake-effect climate. Today, the ridges of the North Shore have by far the highest annual snowfall and longest-lasting snow cover in Minnesota.

There's another reason why cross-country skiing fits this region like a mitten on a ski pole—the people of the North Shore. The history of cross-country skiing is long and mostly Scandinavian. It's no wonder that Minnesota, with its strong Scandinavian heritage, became such a hot spot for "Nordic" skiing.

But where the Swedes and Norwegians settled in the south and west of the state, it was the Finns who came to the North Shore and left their mark. Korkki Nordic Ski Center in rural Duluth was an early center of skiing, with trails built by Charlie Banks in 1954 on land homesteaded by his Finnish father-in-law. A 1977 effort by Governor Rudy Perpich (a native of northeastern Minnesota) to make Minnesota the "Ski Touring Capital of the Nation" resulted in a flurry of activity with new standards, legislation, and trail signage.

North Shore community members were responsible for most of the trails we see today. Local skiers and resort owners, with training from state and national clubs, made up crews that built hundreds, even thousands, of miles of ski trails. Trails such as those at Sugarbush in Tofte were built with collaboration from resort owners, the Forest Service, and local residents. In Duluth, local volunteers joined with the city parks department to lace trails through the city's green spaces. One Finn built his own trails at Piedmont only to have them adopted by the city later on.

Why are these trails so darn good? Because time and nature and people have made it so.

Paying your dues

There is almost no such thing as a free ski outing. Despite the hard work of volunteers, money is always necessary to fuel the chain saws and pay for the grooming equipment. If you find a trail that seems to be free, chances are there is an opportunity for you to help out either financially or physically. The North Shore is blessed with a tremendous wealth of skiing opportunities, thanks to skiers willing to pitch in and help out.

Minnesota state passes. The Great Minnesota Ski Pass is an incredible bargain, and they are required at most of the 35 Minnesota areas described in this book. The pass generates funds through the Department of Natural Resources' Grant-In-Aid program for building, maintaining, and grooming Minnesota ski trails. Passes are available on a daily or yearly basis. (See sidebar on next page for complete details on pass fees and how to purchase them).

Private areas. There are a number of cross-country ski areas in the region that are privately owned and maintained. These areas charge their own usage fees, typically $10 to $18 a day. Often these trail fees are included in the cost of lodging for guests at nearby resorts. Annual and family passes are often available. The Great Minnesota Ski Pass is generally not required at these private areas, but inquire locally to be sure.

For the price of tickets to these private areas, skiers will find consistently well-groomed trails, generally excellent facilities, and a variety of skiing challenges. For the total skiing vacation, these facilities are an excellent choice.

Local clubs. The tradition of volunteering and local involvement has not been lost in the growth of private resorts and the statewide pass. In fact, anywhere you ski there is likely a local group working hard year-round to keep your skiing experience excellent. These groups survive on tiny annual budgets supported mostly by membership contributions.

Since buying and using the statewide pass is such a good bargain, take the time and spend the ten bucks or so to join and support one of these local clubs. Your money will be well spent. A little sweat equity always helps, too; you can donate time in the fall to clear trails, in the winter to fill bare spots, and in the spring to clear debris.

Rules of the road

Regardless of where you ski, some basic rules of courtesy and safety apply.

Follow designated trail directions. This is for your safety and your enjoyment. One-way trails keep skiers from running into each other on hills and blind turns. They also keep skiing parties separate from each other, giving more of a wilderness feel to the experience.

Follow designated trail uses. Many trails are for both skate skiers and classic skiers. Skate skiers should keep their ski tips away from the classic track. Alternately, classic skiers should stay in the tracks and allow skate skiers to pass.

Dogs are not allowed on trails. With a few exceptions, dogs should not be taken on your ski outing. They scare away wildlife and degrade the groomed trail with their feet and their feces. Some ski areas have designated one of their trails for canine use. Other areas designate a day or two each week to bring your dog on the trail. See page 16 for trails that allow dogs.

Fill in "sitzmarks" if you fall. That crater of snow left from your spill will easily lead to another fall for the next skier. Pack in the snow again, run your skis through the groomed track and make it safe again.

Ski under control. If that hill seems too steep for you, snowplow or sidestep down. It is always okay to take off your skis and walk down. This is both for your safety and the safety of the people below.

Do not obstruct the trail. When you take a break, step out of the track so that others can ski by. This is especially important if you are on a hill.

When removing skis and walking, walk on the side of the trail. Try to keep the groomed trail as neat as possible for the next skiers. In general, ski trails should not be used for either snowshoeing or hiking in winter.

THE GREAT MINNESOTA SKI PASS

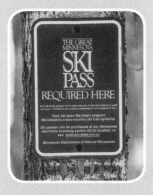

To ski on many public trails, you'll need a Great Minnesota Ski Pass sold by the Department of Natural Resources (DNR). Skiers age 16 and older must have a current ski pass in their possession when skiing on designated trails (or sign it, take a photo of both the front and back sides, and keep a digital copy on your phone). All trail systems in this guide requiring a Great Minnesota Ski Pass are noted in their descriptions.

A one-day pass is $10; a one-year pass is $25; and a three-year pass is $70 (all effective July 1 to June 30, including the purchasing season). The Great Minnesota Ski Pass can be purchased a number of ways:

· **Online**. Visit the DNR at **dnr.state.mn.us/licenses/skipass/index.html**

· **In person.** All Minnesota state parks on the North Shore sell the ski pass, sometimes with a self-service box. You can also visit any Electronic License System vendor, like convenience stores, hardware stores and bait shops. Check the DNR's web site for a location near you.

· **By phone.** Purchase a pass 24 hours/day by calling 888-665-4236. A 3% convenience fee is added to the cost. You'll need a driver's license or state ID and a credit card when calling.

Your Ski Pass will arrive in the mail about two weeks after purchasing online or by phone. But you can still hit the ski trails right away, as you'll receive a purchase confirmation number—write it down and carry it with you until your pass arrives by mail. If you are stopped, verify your ski pass purchase by using that number.

The pass really is required. If caught without one, the penalty is substantial.

A word on trail ratings

The difficulty ratings used in this book for trail descriptions and in trail maps are taken from the original, locally-produced trail maps. There is no standard rating system for ski areas, neither in the names of the levels nor in what they mean. Use the descriptions as provided and where the ratings seem truly inaccurate by this author, the text makes that point.

Some trails are labeled "easy," "easier," "beginner," or marked with a circle. These are suitable for all skiers. The terrain is level; if there are uphills, skiers won't have to "herringbone" for more than a few feet, and any downhill will be easy with a long run-out and no turns.

Some trails are labeled "more difficult," "intermediate," or marked with a square. These trails have some hills. Short uphills require a herringbone climb, and downhills require some ability to turn.

Some trails are labeled "advanced," "expert," "most difficult," or marked with a diamond. These require advanced skills such as snowplow turns and extended herringbone climbing. Expect sharp and steep turns on downhills (including hairpin turns) and long climbs.

Andrew's lists

The following lists are the author's picks for top ski trails on the North Shore...all depending on what you are looking for. If your favorite isn't here, rest easy because absolutely no scientific procedure was applied!

Best grooming. *Here are your best chances for smooth, fresh, and precise grooming regardless of the conditions. Committed groomers come out the first chance they get.*

- Upper Spirit Mountain
- Grand Avenue Nordic Center
- Snowflake Nordic Center
- Boulder Lake
- Korkki Nordic Ski Center
- Sugarbush Trail System
- Pincushion Mountain
- Central Gunflint
- Upper Gunflint

Trails my mother would like. *These have gentle loops, aren't crowded, but have a few easy hills and are scenic.*

- Jay Cooke State Park: CCC Trail
- Superior Municipal Forest: Red Loop
- Biskey Ponds: Wolf Run, Black Spruce trails
- Boulder Lake: Otter Run, Blue Ox trails
- Flathorn-Gegoka Ski Trail: Central Loops
- Cascade River State Park: Cedar Woods
- George Washington Pines
- Central Gunflint: Summer Home Road, Ox Cart trails

Absolutely "free." *These trails have no permits or fees required.*

- Pine Valley Ski Area
- Boulder Lake
- George Washington Pines
- Bagley Nature Area

Most off the beaten path. *Really get away from it all on these trails.*

- Jay Cooke State Park: Spruce, High trails
- Northwoods Ski Touring Trail: Tettegouche Connector
- Tettegouche State Park
- Sugarbush Trail System: Picnic Loop, Sixmile Crossing trails
- Banadad Trail
- Upper Gunflint: Magnetic Rock

Longest season. *Deep snow away from Lake Superior's warmth, plus quality grooming, let you ski early and late.*

- Afterhours Ski Trail
- Piedmont and Hartley Park trails
- Snowflake Nordic Center
- Flathorn-Gegoka Ski Trail
- Sugarbush Trail System: Moose Fence trailhead
- Sugarbush Trail System: Onion River Road trailhead
- Pincushion Mountain
- Central and Upper Gunflint Trails

Best views of Lake Superior. *You might have to work for it, but you'll find great views from high bluffs or the shoreline.*

- Piedmont Trail
- Chester Park Trail

- Gooseberry Falls State Park
- Cascade River State Park: Lakeshore Loop, Moose Mountain trails
- Pincushion Mountain

Most family friendly. *Out for the day? The following offer trails for beginner and advanced skiers, plus warming huts and restrooms.*
- Afterhours Ski Trail
- Jay Cooke State Park
- Superior Municipal Forest
- Grand Avenue Nordic Center
- Snowflake Nordic Center
- Korkki Nordic Ski Center
- Gooseberry Falls State Park
- Cascade River State Park
- Pincushion Mountain

Best downhill routes. *Arrange a car shuttle so you can do these "norpine" trails from ridgeline to lakeshore.*
- Tofte Trail, Sugarbush Trail System
- Caribou Connector (Norpine/Hall-Massie Loop)
- Norpine/Deer Yard to Cascade Lodge
- Bally Creek to Cascade River State Park

Screamers. *These downhill shots take your breath away. When you can't see the bottom from the top, get ready!*
- Upper Spirit Mountain: George Hovland 10K
- Lester Park Trail: Upper Loop side hills
- Korkki Nordic Ski Center: Iso Maki Big Hill
- Gooseberry Falls State Park: Birch Hill loop
- Tettegouche State Park: Lower Loop
- Sugarbush Trail System: Bridge Run
- Central Gunflint: North-South Link, Overlook trails
- Upper Gunflint: West End Trail

Where to ski with your dog. *For all of these dog-friendly trails, your canine companion should be on a leash.*
- Superior Municipal Forest: Blue trails
- Lester Park Trail: Golf Course
- Snowflake Nordic Center: Members only, all trails
- Boulder Lake: Thursdays and Sundays only, all trails

- Biskey Ponds Ski Trail: Wolf Run Trail
- Sugarbush Trail System: Summit View, Maple Loop, Upland Loop trails
- Norpine trails: Whitesides, Deer Track Loop, Cascade Connector
- Bally Creek: Skijoring Trail
- Pincushion Mountain: East Overlook
- George Washington Pines
- Upper Gunflint: Amperage Way

WHICH SKIS, PLEASE?

When you're headed to the North Shore for a ski getaway, what skis should you bring? For many, that's easy: bring the pair you own. However, the wide range of trails, conditions, and topography on the North Shore call out for a little variety in your ski selection.

Wax skis. Waxable skis promise glide, quiet and speed...if you get the waxing right. Wax skis are great when the temps are 28 degrees or below and the snow is fresh, and freshly groomed. Versatile "Swix Blue Extra" wax can take you through almost the entire season here. It takes a few minutes at the trailhead to get the wax applied before you start striding, but for a longer ski outing in primo conditions, it's totally worth it.

No-wax skis. For shorter outings or when the temps are above 30 degrees, no-wax skis promise no-hassle skiing—waxing gets much trickier as the temps climb above 30. No-wax skis are either the old-fashioned fish-scale variety or the new-fangled "skin skis," which have a line of fuzzy grip material right down the middle of the ski. They are especially useful during the warmer and late-season days of February, March, and even April.

Get fitted by a pro. If you are buying equipment, go to a ski shop and get fitted by an expert. A sales pro will ask good questions about how you plan to ski, and they'll make sure you get the right skis for your style and body type. There is no one-size-fits-all in skis; getting a custom solution based on you is often the key to a beautiful cross-country skiing experience. ❋

Duluth-Superior Area

This must be paradise. From anywhere within the city limits of Duluth and Superior, you are never more than a few miles away from terrific skiing. From the wild curves and scenic views of Chester Park, to the backcountry pines and vast variety of Boulder Lake, from the winter camping at Pattison State Park, to the the competitions at Snowflake Nordic Center, the range of options will keep any skier busy all winter long. Plus, from Duluth-Superior you can hit either the north or south shore trails of Lake Superior, depending on where the best snow is found. Some of these trails roll through ballfields and backyards, others take you into wolf country. Whether you're visiting or living here, prepare for great skiing.

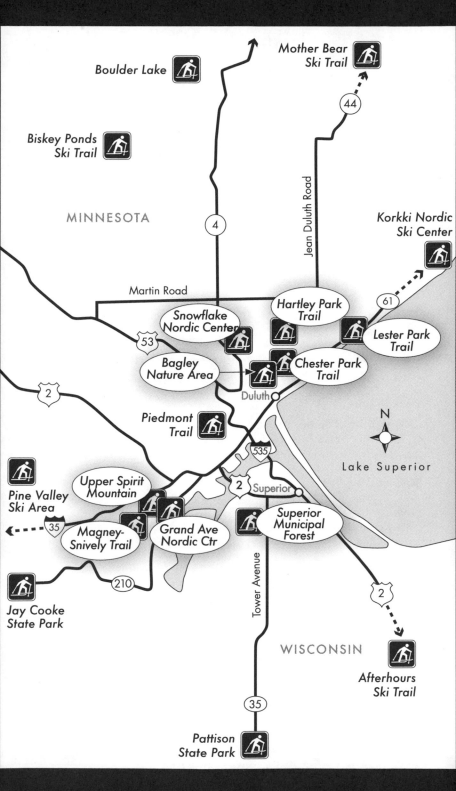

Jay Cooke State Park

Carlton, Minnesota

Trailhead access
Drive three miles east of Carlton on Highway 210 to the "Swinging Bridge" and the River Inn Visitor Center. Or drive from Duluth and Fond du Lac west on Highway 210.

Total groomed trail: 48.1K
Classic skiing: 48.1K

Trail difficulty
Trails range from easy to advanced. Beginning skiers should stay on the north side of the swinging bridge, while advanced skiers have a wide range of terrain. If you're planning on skiing Spruce Trail, the trail on the edge of the system, call the park office ahead of time to see if it's been groomed.

Pass requirements
- Great Minnesota Ski Pass
- Minnesota State Park vehicle permit. Daily permit ($7) or annual permit ($35). Ski passes and vehicle permits are sold in the park office.

Trailhead facilities
State park visitor center with restrooms, vending machines, fireplace.

Snow conditions
dnr.state.mn.us/snow_depth/trails.html?facility_id=4137

What makes it unique
There is an amazing amount of good skiing here within easy access of Duluth. You can walk across a dramatic bridge over the St. Louis River—crossing a rushing river and sharp, 1.6 billion-year-old metamorphic rocks—to reach ski trails on the south side of the park.

Information
Jay Cooke State Park, 218-673-7000
dnr.state.mn.us/parkfinder/index.html

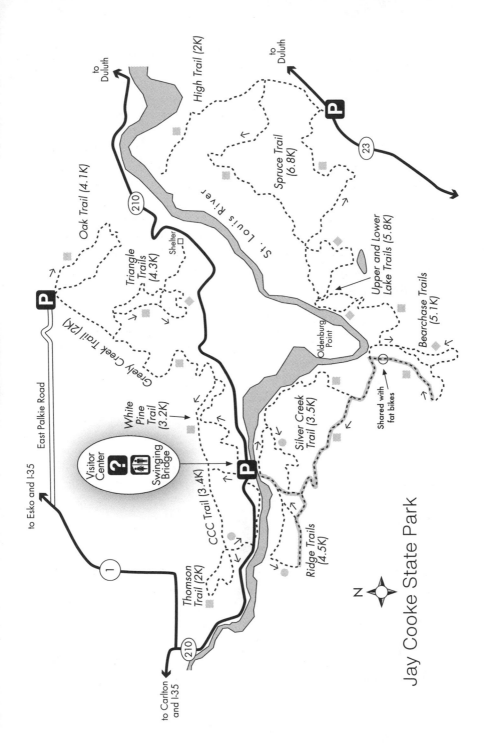

Jay Cooke State Park

South of swinging bridge

One challenging aspect of skiing these trails is getting across the bridge and up the first hill. Most people walk across the bridge and up the first hill. A little extra work to reach these trails gives you solitude and adventure.

RIDGE TRAILS (4.5K)

Easier. As the name implies, the east and west Ridge Trails traverse a ridge above the St. Louis River; the ridge is thick with maples. With three smaller loops, this section is perfect for goofing around with young kids, if they can get there. Parts of this trail are shared with fat bikes.

SILVER CREEK AND BEAR CHASE TRAILS (8.6K)

Intermediate and advanced. These trails begin to take you into the back country of the park. From here on, the farther you go, the fewer people you will see. From the bridge, the Silver Creek Trail is a 5K loop along the edge of the river valley with great views, returning along Silver Creek's wetlands back to the Ridge Trails. As long as you've come this far, cross Silver Creek and take the Bear Chase Trails, too; the trails take you up tight valleys then down narrow ridges for a fun, advanced ride. Parts of these trails are shared with fat bikes.

UPPER AND LOWER LAKE TRAILS (5.8K)

Advanced. These advanced trails will keep you huffing and puffing as you climb from the banks of the St. Louis River 200 feet up and glide back down again. These and the following trails are not groomed as often as the inner trails, so you should check with the park ranger before heading out here for the day. Watch out on steep, two-way trails.

SPRUCE AND HIGH TRAILS (8.8K)

Intermediate. Once past the advanced Lower and Upper Lake trails, you'll enter more level, intermediate country—and you're almost guaranteed to have it all to yourself. The Spruce Trail itself is a 6.8K loop through cedar, pines, and maple, with the southern half having constant views off the bluff; if that's not enough, take the High Trail 2K to an overlook of the St. Louis River. You can also access these trails from a small parking area on Highway 23.

North of swinging bridge

The trails north of the bridge start from the parking lot on the opposite side of the park office. Most skiers walk the thirty yards to Highway 210 and cross it before putting on their skis.

CCC TRAIL (3.4K)

Easier. This trail takes old roadways through relatively open terrain around the campground. The eastern half in particular is very easy going after the first climb. The western half gets trickier when the trail leaves the old roadway and winds down to cross Highway 210. The return along the river bank is scenic any time of year.

WHITE PINE TRAIL (3.2K)

Intermediate. This is a delightful loop through dense groves of white pine and a maple ridgeline. The first 0.4K follows an old roadbed downhill; the trail turns left off the old road and starts climbing for a long herringbone up and around to a shelter with a great view of the St. Louis River valley. Enjoy a snack here as you take off for a day's ski. The trail winds through some rolling terrain on the south side, then levels out on the north side. Some of the turns are tricky here, so be prepared for quick moves.

THOMSON TRAIL (2K)

Intermediate. This trail is made "intermediate" by a long, moderate climb and daring swoop down and up past large white pines. Otherwise, this is mostly level terrain through open, deciduous woods.

GREELY CREEK TRAIL (2K)

Intermediate. This trail connects the Oldenburg Point trails and the White Pine trails with the Triangle and Oak loops. The trail gives you a close-up look at the Thomson hydropower operations of Minnesota Power as it follows power lines and then skirts the shore of Forbay Lake before crossing over the top of the small dam.

TRIANGLE TRAILS (4.3K)

Intermediate to advanced. Noticeably more difficult than the Oak Trails, this 2.2K loop rolls through a variety of forests, with a spur to a shelter.

The 1.3K advanced side trail, which dips off the plateau and into the hillside, is pretty wild and may not be groomed.

OAK TRAIL (4.1K)

Intermediate. Access this loop from the Greely Creek Trail or more commonly from Palkie Road, 1.6 miles east of County Road 1. This trail is remarkably level as it curves around the rim of a plateau. As the name implies, there are lots of oak here, plus some great views to distant ridges.

SHIVER LIKE A CHICKADEE

The black-capped chickadee has a "bundle" of survival tricks, including... "bundling." On cold nights, chickadees will gather in a flock of about six birds and bundle together in the hole of an evergreen tree, keeping each other warm through the night. The chickadees will go into a sort of torpor, letting their body temperatures drop as much as 12° C. They maintain this temperature all night, through outbreaks of group shivering.

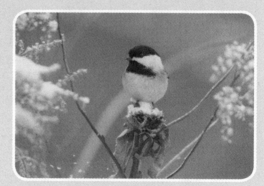

Next time you're out with a group and it's getting cold, be like the chickadee: get a group hug going and have everybody shimmy to stay toasty!

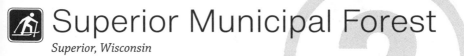

Superior Municipal Forest

Superior, Wisconsin

Trailhead access

There are two trailheads: **(1)** Take 28th Street one mile west from Tower Avenue. Parking lot is on south side of road, marked with a sign; or **(2)** Continue on 28th Street until it turns into Billings Drive. Follow Billings Drive for about two miles to the parking lot on the left with the ski trail signage.

Total groomed trail: 26K

Classic skiing: 26K   Skate skiing: 26K

Trail difficulty

Beginners should stick to the 28th Street trailhead, with the easier trails. Advanced skiers will enjoy the Billings Drive trailhead, with quick access to the physically challenging Yellow Loop.

Pass requirements

- City of Superior day passes ($5) and season passes ($20-$30) available at trailheads and at Northwest Outlet in Superior. Passes required for ages 16 and older; senior (age 65) discount available.

Trailhead facilities

Restrooms and warming hut at 28th Street trailhead. Toilet at Billings Drive trailhead.

Snow conditions

Frequent reports on skinnyski.com

What makes it unique

A wide variety of terrain is found in the country's second largest municipal forest. The system is ranked as one of Wisconsin's best cross-country ski trails. The trails are groomed quite wide, giving both skate skiers and classic skiers plenty of room.

Information

Superior Parks and Recreation Department, 715-395-7270
ci.superior.wi.us

RED TRAILS—INNER AND OUTER (3K)

Easy. This is a wide and level warm-up trail, great for families and first-time skiers. Towering pines give this loop a cozy feel. Both the inner and outer trail lead from one "island" of white pines to another; these "islands" are on ground that is just a few feet higher than the "sea" of alder, which are on lower, wetter ground.

BLUE TRAIL (2K)

Advanced. There are so many fun ups and downs on this trail it feels much longer than 2K. Boreal forest and wild hills distinguish this short section from the rest of the trails in the Superior Municipal Forest. Take counterclockwise.

GREEN TRAILS (INNER AND OUTER) (5K)

Intermediate. This network of trails runs through fields and open woods, zooming down to cross the occasional stream and then up the other side. Most skiers take these trails counterclockwise (as indicated by the arrows posted on the trails). The trails on the north and west sides take you into more ambitious terrain, with steep hills and sharp turns, but for the most part this is family-friendly and fun.

YELLOW LOOP (10K)

Advanced. Access this trail from the Billings Drive trailhead. There are some serious downhills followed by grunting uphills on the eastern side of the loop, as the trail descends into valleys of the streams that empty into the St. Louis River estuary. Almost all of these downward swoops can be bypassed with side loops. Take the Cedar Point spur trail and you can get out onto Kimball's Bay. Settle into a Zen-like groove on the return side of the loop, as the terrain and forest hardly changes for over 2K.

PURPLE TRAIL (4.8K PLUS 1.3K CUT-OFF)

More difficult. You can either park at the Billings Drive trailhead for this loop or reach it from the main trailhead via the Green trail. The main "Outer" loop is meant to be taken clockwise. You'll ski about 3K through mature pine and hardwood forest with no bothersome trail intersections (from S to W). The terrain overall is flat as a pancake, but there are four or five major downhill swoops, each followed by a steep climb back up to the

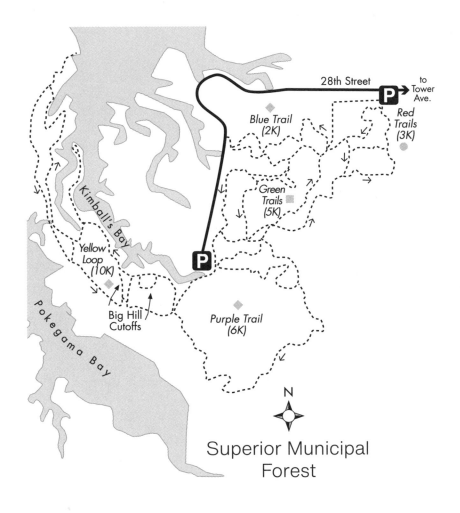

28th Street

to Tower Ave.

Blue Trail (2K)

Red Trails (3K)

Kimball's Bay

Green Trails (5K)

Yellow Loop (10K)

Big Hill Cutoffs

Purple Trail (6K)

Pokegama Bay

N

Superior Municipal Forest

flats. The last kilometer, from W back to X, is shared with a snowmobile trail for a swoop down to Kimball's Bay. If you're not up for the steep descents and climbs, there's a cut-off from S back to the trailhead at X, making a 2.5K "Inner" loop.

Pattison State Park
Superior, Wisconsin

Trailhead access
Drive 12 miles south of Superior on Highway 35 (not Interstate 35). Take park road toward campground and continue driving to ski trailhead.

Total groomed trail: 7K
Classic skiing: 7K

Trail difficulty
Like a lot of trail systems, the further out you get, the more challenging the trails are. All but beginner skiers can easily do all the trails here in an hour or two.

Pass requirements
- Wisconsin state park vehicle permit. Daily permits ($8 Wisconsin residents, $11 non-Wisconsin residents) and annual permits ($28 Wisconsin residents, $38 non-Wisconsin residents) available; senior discount offered (age 65). Available at park office, online, or at 888-305-0398.

Trailhead facilities
Restroom at park office.

Snow conditions
dnr.wi.gov/TrailConditions

What makes it unique
This trail system gives you a taste of a different forest type than you'd find on the North Shore. Large basswoods and oaks mix in with stands of maple. Pattison picks up some lake-effect snow, so you may find better conditions here than in Duluth. For an extra adventure, ski in to the campsites on the Oak Ridge Trail for a night of winter camping. Check at the park office for details.

Information
Pattison State Park, Wisconsin Department of Natural Resources
dnr.wisconsin.gov/topic/parks/pattison/recreation/winter

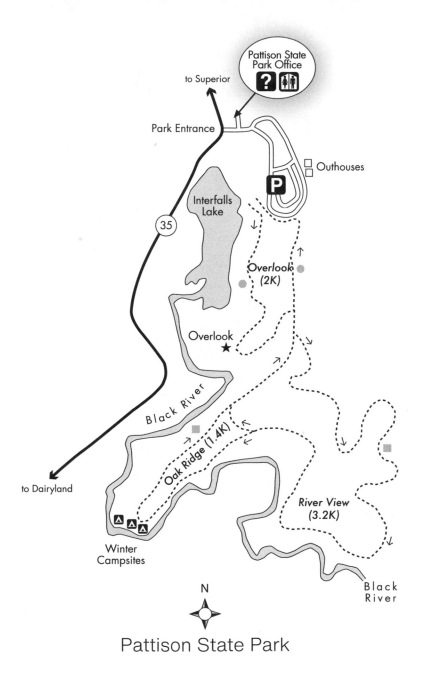

Pattison State Park

OVERLOOK (2K)

Easier. This mostly level loop starts off near an historic forestry facility, passes maintenance buildings, then enters a nice maple and oak forest. At the halfway point, there is an overlook of the Black River valley.

RIVER VIEW (3.2K)

Intermediate. This winding, relatively easy loop takes you clockwise through a quiet and remote corner of the park. The last half of the loop runs along the Black River, with nice views of the river. Watch for extra large yellow birch and white pine trees along the trail. Trail runs past an 1880s logging camp.

OAK RIDGE (1.4K)

Intermediate. This short loop has plenty of turns and short hills through pockets of birch and fir. A shelter at the far end of the loop marks the entrance to three backpack campsites on the Black River just above Little Manitou Falls (there are outhouses available by the campsites). These are used infrequently in winter.

POPPING BIRCHES

It's a cold you can feel deep in your body, your breath sending icy knives into the recesses of your lungs. Luckily, it's just a short walk up the driveway before turning in. A dangerous cold, with the night sky so starry you know it will get even colder. Tonight will be a far cry from the warmth of the afternoon, when winter sun warmed the hillsides and the birch trees, melting the sap within. Now,

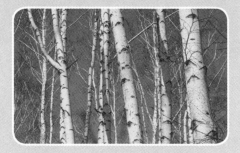

with the return of the real cold, the sap freezes again—and freezes fast. The freezing sap expands and cracks open the side of the birch with a muffled gunshot. You think "what's that?" and then you remember: it's February, the Moon of the Popping Trees. ❄

Afterhours Ski Trail

Brule, Wisconsin

Trailhead access
On U.S. Highway 2, 30 miles east of Superior, Wisconsin at the edge of the South Shore snow belt. Just west of downtown Brule, turn south on Afterhours Road directly into the parking lot.

Total groomed trail: 23.4K
Classic skiing: 23.4K   Skate skiing: 20.8K

Trail difficulty
Mostly intermediate terrain is found here. Trails are groomed quite wide, so only the steepest hills and turns down by the river present a real challenge.

Pass Requirements
- Wisconsin State Trail Pass. Annual ($25) and daily ($5) passes sold at the trailhead. Under 16 ski free. The Brule Valley Ski Club works with Brule River State Forest to maintain and improve the trail system. The club welcomes annual memberships; look for details at the trailhead.

Trailhead facilities
Heated shelter, outhouse. The town of Brule has restaurants, gas stations, and a motel.

Snow conditions
brulexcski.com/trail-condition

What makes it unique
If you want to ski the North Shore but all the snow has fallen on the South Shore, this is your easiest opportunity to enjoy lake-effect snowbelt skiing. Duluth can be totally brown, but as you drive east past Poplar and Maple, suddenly the snow piles up. Here, early season skiing can start in mid-November.

Information
Brule River State Forest, 715-372-5678, brulexcski.com
wisconsintrailguide.com/cross-country-skiing/afterhours.html

ENTRY AND RETURN (2.3K)

Beginner and advanced. Choices, choices. Easy start or hard? Easy return or difficult? Everyone starting these trails makes these choices right away, but both trails roll up through white pine to the same spot, Hilltop Junction, then onto the triangle trails that connect to the Loop trail. On the way back, it's the classic end-of-ski downhill run, either easy or difficult—but both fun.

MAPLE (1.4K)

Beginner. Gentle curves take you through sugar maple forest.

SALLY'S CLASSIC (6.9K)

Intermediate. Weaving through the western half of the system, this narrow, singe-track trail gives classic skiers their own delightful loop. In certain conditions, this is the best skiing at After Hours. Beginner skiers, watch out for a hidden steep downhill about a kilometer past the major Six Corners junction.

BALSAM (0.7K)

Beginner. Consider this the access trail to the 3.1K Loop.

ASPEN (1.1K)

Beginner. This is the main one-way trail taking you back to the trailhead. It's curvy but easy. Take it after the Spruce Trail for a beginner route.

SPRUCE (1.4K)

Beginner. Nice flat trail that is lined with the distinctive Norway spruce, an exotic tree noted for its drooping branches. This connects with the Entry and Aspen trails for a fun beginner route of about 4K.

OAK (3.5K)

Intermediate. Starts easy and flat, following an unplowed, summer-only road straight to the west. Things get interesting when you finally turn left, crossing wetland areas, passing large Norway spruce, and winding back down toward the Brule River valley.

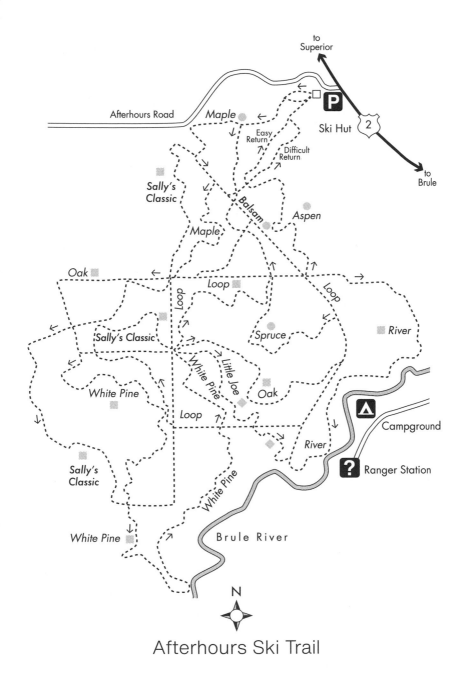

Afterhours Ski Trail

RIVER (2.2K)

Intermediate. When the snow is fresh, this is considered the best trail in the system—with great downhill runs, views of the Brule River, and maybe even wolf scat near the tracks. The pine forest can leave needles on the trail. This is the route of an 1890s logging railroad and was the route used by early Brule River vacationers to reach their camps.

WHITE PINE (4.2K)

Intermediate. This is a long, winding trail that starts in white pines and descends toward the river valley into open aspen woods. Take a break at the old, gnarled jack pine overlooking the Brule River valley before starting the gentle climb back up.

LOOP (3.1K)

Intermediate. This is signed as "North Loop," "West Loop," "South Loop" and "East Loop," but it's all one trail, mostly flat, easy and wide. Near the "Northeast Junction" is an unmarked outhouse.

LITTLE JOE (1.2K)

Advanced. This is rated advanced because of the wild roller coaster near its end at the River Trail by the Little Joe Rapids lookout. It feels like running a slalom course, with large white pines as the slalom gates.

GREAT SNACKS FOR YOUR PACK

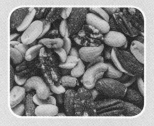

What's compact, hard to break, won't freeze, and is full of complex carbohydrates? The ideal trail snack, that's what! For outings longer than an hour, pack away some extra fuel like raisins, peanuts or their yogurt-covered cousins. Hard cheeses hold up well, but slice them before you head out. For a trail lunch, nothing's more delicious than a bagel with meat or cheese. Don't bother with anything wrapped up like chocolate candies; you'll be a litterbug for sure. Also, keep a water bottle inside your pack to prevent it from freezing. ❄

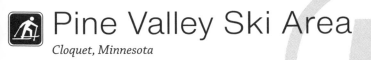

Pine Valley Ski Area

Cloquet, Minnesota

Trailhead access
From Highway 33 (the main strip off Interstate 35), turn west on Armory Drive by the McDonalds. After a short 0.2 miles, turn left at the fork to Olympic Drive. Head around to the left side of the Arena to the large parking area for Pine Valley Park.

Total groomed trail: 6K
Classic skiing: 6K   Lighted trail: 2.5K

Trail difficulty
The entire system is intermediate, with some long climbs and challenging turns.

Pass requirements
• None

Trailhead facilities
Outhouses

Snow conditions
facebook.com/pinevalley360

What makes it unique
Just minutes from the commercial strip of Cloquet and right next to the high school hockey arena, Pine Valley Park is a community hub that happens to have a great ski trail. One of Minnesota's last Nordic Combined centers, there is an active ski jump in addition to the cross-country trails.

Information
Pine Valley Ski Area, 218-269-2948
facebook.com/CloquetSkiClub

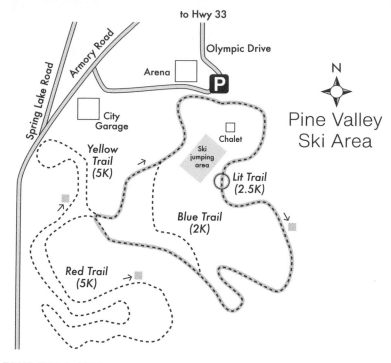

BLUE TRAIL (2K)

Intermediate. This is the innermost of three nested loops. Convenient directional signs with color-coded arrows make it easy to sort out the three colored loops. The trail begins under the park's tall pines. The trail does a long climb up and around to the top of the ski jump hill, then rolls through a wooded valley before returning on an unlit cut-off trail to the chalet area.

YELLOW TRAIL (3.5K, 2.5K LIT)

Intermediate. The Yellow Trail continues past the Blue Trail cut-off; this adds about another 2K to the Blue Trail. There's a busy trail junction called "Lee's Crossing" where the 2.5K lit loop cuts off to the right. The final leg of the Yellow Trail is narrower and a fun downhill run.

RED TRAIL (5K)

Intermediate. The Red Trail adds another 1.5K on to the Yellow Trail. This wider, rolling trail provides a more mellow cruising experience but is still considered intermediate. There may be a narrow, seldom-used connection with a multi-use trail known as the White Pine Loop.

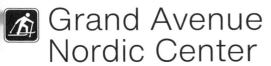

Grand Avenue Nordic Center

Duluth, Minnesota

Trailhead access

About two miles west of Interstate 35 on Grand Avenue, watch for entrance on right to Spirit Mountain and the Grand Avenue Chalet. Be sure you're not navigating to Upper Spirit Mountain.

Total groomed trail: 2.5K

Classic skiing: 2.5K   Skate skiing: 2.5K

Trail difficulty

You'll find easier to more difficult skiing here. Trails are wide and the turns are forgiving.

Pass requirements

• Daily pass ($10 individual/$5 student) available at trailhead chalet. Children under age 6 free. Season passes with early bird discount available online.

Trailhead facilities

Full chalet with changing areas, bathrooms, restaurant, and bar.

Snow conditions

Visit spiritmt.com and look for the Mountain Message

What makes it unique

Nordic skiing advocates in Duluth have come together to plan and fund what will be a state-of-the-art cross-county ski center. The long-term vision includes additional trail with snow making and lights, plus a connector to the Upper Spirit Mountain trails. Currently, the snow making on 1.5K provides reliable early-season skiing.

Information

Spirit Mountain, spiritmt.com/nordic-center-trail-system
Duluth Cross-Country Ski Club, duluthxc.com/grand-avenue-nordic-center

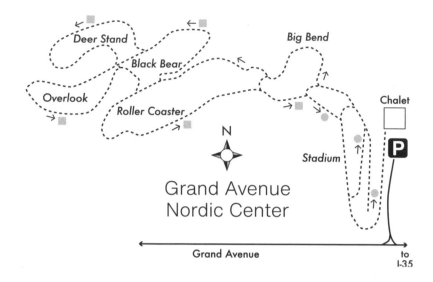

STADIUM AREA (0.6K)

Easier. Partially lit. Wide-open field between the Chalet and the trails, built for mass starts and dramatic race finishes. Though rated Easier, it's all either a gradual up or a gentle rolling down.

BIG BEND AND ROLLER COASTER (1.5K)

Intermediate. Ski up through pines and hardwoods and cross the historic Duluth, Winnipeg and Pacific railroad bed. As you climb, you might notice downhill skiers nearby, a reminder that you're climbing. A lot. There's a short level stretch followed by the roller coaster descent.

BLACK BEAR AND OVERLOOK (0.6K)

Intermediate. Combine these two small loops into one and you get a long climb followed by the longest level stretch in the whole system. You'll need a good snowplow turn to get around the hairpin descent, then be sure to catch the brief open view of broad Spirit Lake. As of 2021, snow making only covered the Black Bear half.

DEER STAND (0.3K)

Intermediate. Another steep climb, followed by a short level area, closing with a curving down hill. As of 2021, there was no snow making here.

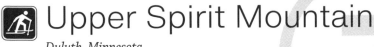

Upper Spirit Mountain

Duluth, Minnesota

Trailhead access
Take Skyline Drive from Interstate 35 (Exit #249) and follow signs to Spirit Mountain Recreation Area. Stay on Skyline Drive past entrance to downhill ski area on left. Watch for turn on right side marked for the campground and Nordic center.

Total groomed trail: 16K
Classic skiing: 16K   Skate skiing: 16K

Pass requirements
- Daily pass ($10 individual/$5 student) available at trailhead chalet. Children under age 6 free. Season passes with early bird discount available online.

Trail difficulty
This system is best for intermediate and advanced skiers. Most of the trails, even The 3K beginner trail, are reached by an access trail that would be rated intermediate. Real beginners can use the 1K Campground Loop.

Trailhead facilities
Chalet, restrooms

Snow conditions
Frequent reports on skinnyski.com

What makes it unique
This trail system is maintained by volunteers from the Duluth Cross Country Ski Club (or DXC) and it often provides the best and most consistent skiing conditions in Duluth. The presence of these ski trails and extensive old-growth forest helped to stop a proposed golf course development here.

Information
Duluth Cross-Country Ski Club, duluthxc.com
spiritmt.com/nordic-center-trail-system

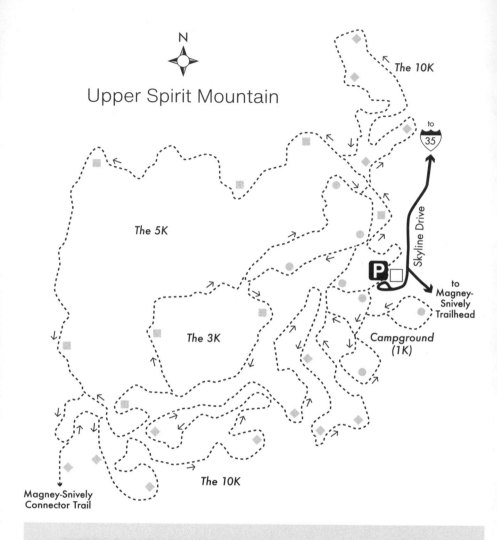

N

Upper Spirit Mountain

The 10K

to
35

Skyline Drive

The 5K

P

to
Magney-
Snively
Trailhead

The 3K

Campground
(1K)

The 10K

Magney-Snively
Connector Trail

ONE SKI HILL, TWO XC TRAILS

At Spirit Mountain Recreation Area, there are two distinct cross-country trail systems. **Upper Spirit Mountain** relies on natural snow, and its 16K of trails are managed by the Duluth Cross Country Ski Club. **Grand Avenue Nordic Center** is at the base of the ski hill and has just 2.5K of trails, but these trails benefit from snowmaking machines and lights for night skiing. Long-range plans call for a trail to link the two systems. For now, you can buy a combined season pass that allows you to enjoy both areas. ❄

CAMPGROUND LOOP (1K)

Easier. This easy loop through the campground starts on a wide road, then swoops down and ends with gradual downhills. Some of the best early-season skiing in Duluth is here, with a wide smooth surface.

THE 3K (2.7K)

Easier and more difficult. Most of the loop trails, including this one, start or end at an abandoned shack that you reach with a short, steep climb from the Nordic Center Chalet. The first half of the loop is 1.4K and labeled easier, but there is a long, challenging uphill climb about two-thirds of the way around that is too much for most beginners. The second half of the loop is labeled more difficult, which is accurate.

THE 5K (5.4K)

More difficult. This is a classic intermediate trail, perfectly paced with curvy downhills and uphills just long enough to make you short of breath. After an uninterrupted 2+K in hardwood forests, the trail joins the second half of The 3K back to the abandoned shack where you started.

THE 10K (11K with all the advanced loops)

Most difficult. This trail combines most of The 5K with four advanced loops that wind through steep terrain. It's for the ambitious, experienced skier and seems to get steeper and more curvy as it goes. Save enough energy to whoop and holler at "Omagod" hill. The first advanced loop of 1.8K spins off just past the abandoned shack, the rest come after 2.1K on the intermediate trail. The 1K Magney-Snively Connector trail links Spirit Mountain trails with the rugged city park trails of Magney-Snively,

MOUNTAIN VILLAS AT SPIRIT MOUNTAIN

Octagonal villas are located trailside and slopeside at Spirit Mountain, and four villas are adjacent to the upper Spirit Nordic trails. Information and reservations: **mtvillas.com**

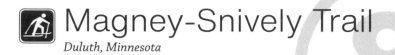

Magney-Snively Trail
Duluth, Minnesota

Trailhead access
Take Interstate 35 to Boundary Avenue exit. Drive 2.5 miles on Skyline Parkway (past Spirit Mountain recreation area), following the road signs for "Magney Ski Area." Parking lot is on left side at end of plowed road; trailhead is on right side of road.

Total groomed trail: 13K
Classic skiing: 13K   Skate skiing: 13K

Trail difficulty
Magney Ski Area has long, challenging loops, difficult both for the hills and turns but also for their length. Although groomed and designated for skating, the trail is narrow and tracked at the far edge, so classic skiers should watch out for overhanging branches.

Pass requirements
• Great Minnesota Ski Pass

Trailhead facilities
None

Snow conditions
City of Duluth Parks & Rec hotline: 218-730-4321, press 1

What makes it unique
The extensive old-growth maple forest and remote-feeling terrain give this in-town ski area a terrific wilderness feel. Long stretches of trail with no junctions to puzzle out make this a true skiing adventure. If you combine all three loops into one big trip, it's 12 kilometers of skiing through Duluth's finest natural area.

Information
City of Duluth Parks and Recreation, 218-730-4300
duluthmn.gov/parks/trails-bikeways/cross-country-ski-trails

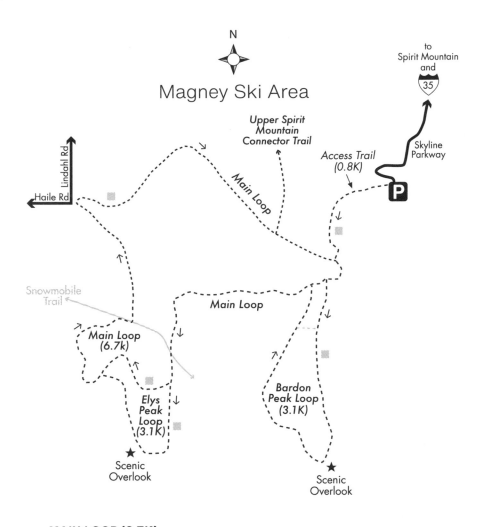

MAIN LOOP (6.7K)

Intermediate. After a 0.8K uphill ski on the access trail, you enter the most wild, natural and remote of Duluth's ski trails. The trail is marked by long, sometimes steep climbs and smooth, glorious downhills.

The second half of the loop includes some beautiful lowland meadows and a massive rock outcrop looming above the trail. The final 2K feature four significant climbs followed by challenging descents. Near the end of the loop, there's a junction for a groomed connector trail that leads to the Upper Spirit Mountain trails.

ELYS PEAK LOOP (3.1K)

Intermediate. Most skiers here continue off the Main Loop for this extra challenge. Although rated intermediate, these are definitely advanced trails: be ready for sharp, downhill turns. The loop leads to an overlook of the beautiful valley below and to a view of Elys Peak, a half mile to the south.

BARDON PEAK LOOP (3.1K)

Intermediate. Soon after joining the main loop from the 0.8K access trail, you will reach the Bardon Peak Loop juncture. This loop and its tremendous overlook offers a view of Duluth, Superior, and the St. Louis River valley below. Climb up into maple woods and descend into ash swamps before rejoining the main trail. If you liked it the first time, do it again!

DULUTH'S FABULOUS CITY PARKS

Magney-Snively, Piedmont, Chester Park, Hartley Park, and Lester Park ski trails

Scattered across the rugged hills of Duluth are some of the finest urban ski trails anywhere, period. Five city parks with 47 kilometers of groomed trails await your sampling, ranging from the short-but-sweet racer's loop at Chester Park to the diverse network of trails at Lester Park; from the backcountry of Magney-Snively to the your-own-backyard atmosphere of Piedmont.

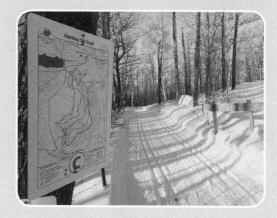

Grooming is regular and professional. For the latest grooming update, call the hotline at 218-730-4321 before heading out to ski or check online at Skinnyski.com, where you're sure to find reviews on current conditions. The trailheads have few facilities, but are all within a mile of whatever you might need. ❆

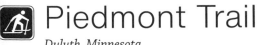

Piedmont Trail

Duluth, Minnesota

Trailhead access
From the stoplight on U.S. 53, take Piedmont Avenue two blocks and turn left on Hutchinson Road. Take Hutchinson Road 0.7 miles uphill to parking lot on the left side of road, near the corner of Adirondack Street.

Total groomed trail: 6K
Classic skiing: 6K

Trail difficulty
The main loop here attracts mostly families and friends, enjoying the relatively easy double set of tracks with fun and conversation. The Expert Loop and the trail beyond the "Chicken Loop Cut-Off" are definitely for more advanced skiers.

Pass requirements
• Great Minnesota Ski Pass

Trailhead facilities
None

Snow conditions
City of Duluth Parks & Rec hotline: 218-730-4321, press 1

What makes it unique
This trail has homespun flavor and character. It was built by Piedmont resident Jerry Nowak, and then turned over to the City of Duluth for management. The clever signs along the trail keep you laughing, and the in-town ease of getting here makes for a quick and satisfying lunchtime fitness break.

Information
City of Duluth Parks and Recreation, 218-730-4300
duluthmn.gov/parks/trails-bikeways/cross-country-ski-trails

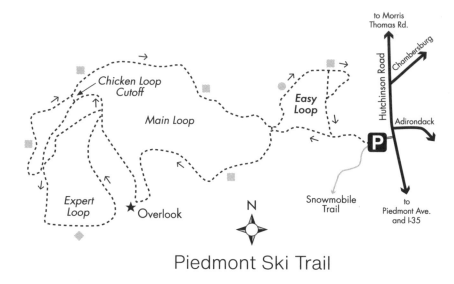

Piedmont Ski Trail

EASY LOOP (1.2K)

Easier/skating and classic. You'll see all types of skiers here. First-timers cling to the sides of the trail practicing their first strides. Confident classic skiers kick and glide through to the longer trails beyond. Skaters are infrequent here and they have a wide middle lane. It's a good loop for a beginner, with a few longer and forgiving downhill runs.

MAIN LOOP (2.8K)

More difficult/classic only. Clever signs urge you on past small dips through a mixed deciduous forest as you climb very gradually to a dramatic overlook, one of the best on Duluth trails. The trail is generally well-suited for beginners except for a short, steep climb known as "Powder Puff-Puff." A fun and more advanced loop at the end can be bypassed by taking a 50-foot cutoff ("Chicken Loop").

EXPERT LOOP (1.1K)

Most difficult/classic only. This loop provides about 1K of steep hills and sharp turns. Snow conditions on this loop can be marginal. The loop is marked by one particularly steep downhill with a blind curve. Many intermediate skiers skip the steep hill and curve, and instead ski from the "E" junction to "F" on an easier 0.3K leg of this trail, rejoining the Main Loop at "F."

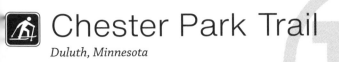

Chester Park Trail
Duluth, Minnesota

Trailhead access
Take Skyline Parkway to the Chester Bowl Ski Area, either east from Kenwood Avenue or west from College Street and 19th Avenue East.

Total groomed trail: 3K
Classic skiing: 3K   Skate skiing: 3K

Trail difficulty
Chester Park is best enjoyed by advanced skiers. Screaming downhill runs with tight turns can include dog walkers, footprint divots, and other trail obstacles, so it's good to keep control of your speed.

Pass requirements
• Great Minnesota Ski Pass

Trailhead facilities
Chalet and restrooms open weekends and some evenings.

Snow conditions
City of Duluth Parks & Rec hotline: 218-730-4321, press 1

What makes it unique
This is a wild and woolly, in-town ski area specifically for advanced skiers and racers. With downhill ski runs and a chairlift in the park, Chester Park can be a complete ski destination.

Information
City of Duluth Parks and Recreation, 218-730-4300.
duluthmn.gov/parks/trails-bikeways/cross-country-ski-trails

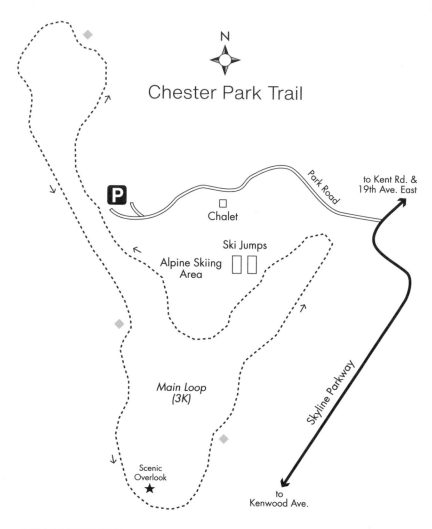

N

Chester Park Trail

P

to Kent Rd. &
19th Ave. East

Park Road

Chalet

Ski Jumps

Alpine Skiing
Area

Skyline Parkway

Main Loop
(3K)

Scenic
Overlook
★

to
Kenwood Ave.

MAIN LOOP (3K)

Advanced. This is designed for advanced skiers, with serious downhills and turns. After a level start, you will cross Chester Creek and start on a roller coaster, up and down and around tight corners. About halfway is a field with a 120° view of Lake Superior. After the field, descend into the forest before one last climb up above the Chester Bowl chairlift for a final run back to where you began, three hairy kilometers before. You may be sharing it with dog walkers, despite signs that prohibit dogs.

Hartley Park Trail
Duluth, Minnesota

Trailhead access
There are three trailheads: **(1)** Use Hartley Nature Center parking lot off Woodland Avenue; **(2)** Take Fairmont Street two blocks west off of Woodland Avenue; or **(3)** Take Hartley Road 0.3 miles from the four-way stop at Arrowhead Road.

Total groomed trail: 5K
Classic skiing: 5K

Trail difficulty
This can be a great trail for a family outing, but parents skiing with children should familiarize themselves with the trail layout beforehand.

Pass requirements
• Great Minnesota Ski Pass

Trailhead facilities
Restrooms at Nature Center.

Snow conditions
City of Duluth Parks & Rec hotline: 218-730-4321, press 1

What makes it unique
Nicely wooded, double-tracked, classic-only trails are a cozy alternative to other Duluth trails. The deep, shady woods tend to hold on well to late-season snow. On Saturdays, you can use the warm restrooms at Hartley Nature Center.

Information
City of Duluth Parks and Recreation, 218-730-4300. duluthmn.gov/parks/trails-bikeways/cross-country-ski-trails

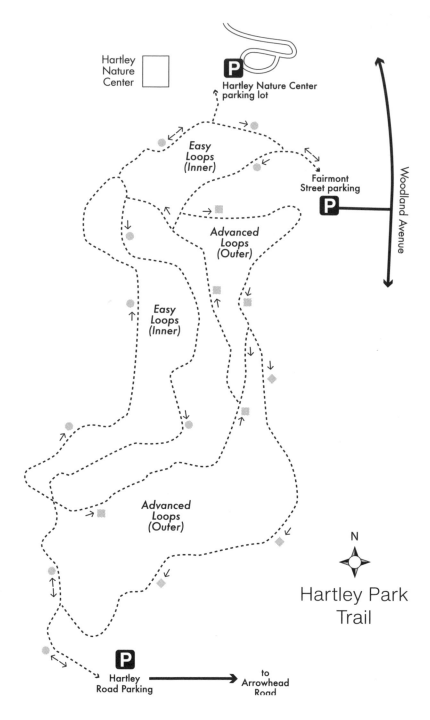

Hartley
Nature
Center

Hartley Nature Center
parking lot

Easy
Loops
(Inner)

Fairmont
Street parking

Woodland Avenue

Advanced
Loops
(Outer)

Easy
Loops
(Inner)

Advanced
Loops
(Outer)

N

Hartley Park
Trail

Hartley
Road Parking

to
Arrowhead
Road

EASY LOOPS (Inner loops) (2.1K to 2.6K)

Easier. From any of the three trailheads, you can follow easier trails around the woods of Hartley Park. But pay attention to the maps and signage, it's easy to get turned around here, and large leftover signs still refer to the Inner and Outer loops which no longer exist. The heart of these easy trails is a 1.6K loop. On both sides of the loop you'll find at least one short uphill climb that will challenge beginners.

ADVANCED LOOPS (Outer loops) (3.1K to 3.6K)

More difficult/most difficult. From any of the three trailheads, take a short stretch of easier trails to reach a 2.4K advanced loop in the core of the Hartley ski trail network. The west side of this loop is a classic intermediate trail with long climbs and some downhill turns. The east side has a long steep initial climb and then rolls around, ending at a challenging, curving downhill. There's a cut-across about halfway along if you want to avoid the hardest part of the loop. Pro-tip: watch for an unmarked right turn near the end of the west side, where you can take a 50-yard shortcut against the grain from I to F.

A NORTHERN SKIER'S CALENDAR

November: Watch the forecast—you might get lucky late in the month, especially inland and on ridgeline areas where early snow sticks first. Skiers often trek to local golf courses in search of skiing.

December: Grooming starts in earnest when snowfall is consistent.

January: It's often cold, but usually snowy. Martin Luther King holiday weekend is busy with skiers on the North Shore.

February: This is peak skiing time, especially over the Presidents' Day weekend when trailside lodging will be fully booked in advance.

March: Afternoons turn warm and start to melt the snow; bring no-wax skis if you have them. There is often a mid- to late-morning magic hour when the temperature rises above freezing and before it turns too warm, when the snow is soft but not too wet. March cross-country skiing conditions are often fabulous.

April: Grooming's over, but there could still be snow in shady areas. The Onion River Road in the Sugarbush Trail System is often one of the last skiable trails on the North Shore. Skiers also seek out still-frozen inland lakes for good skating conditions, often during the colder morning hours. ❄

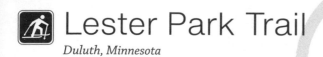

Lester Park Trail
Duluth, Minnesota

Trailhead access
There are four trailheads: **(1)** Take Lester River Road 100 yards up from Superior Street to large parking lot on left; **(2)** Take Seven Bridges Road (Occidental Boulevard) to roadside parking about one mile from Superior Street; **(3)** On Seven Bridges Road, drive farther uphill to the Lester-Amity Chalet parking area on right; or **(4)** Take Lester River Road about 0.5 mile past Trailhead 1 to the golf course on the right.

Total groomed trail: 16.8K
Classic skiing: 16.8K   Skate skiing: 16.8K   Lighted trail: 6K

Trail difficulty
There's a bit of everything here. Everyone starts with the easier Inner Loops, but the upper loops provide real challenge, especially with all the side loop options.

Pass requirements
• Great Minnesota Ski Pass

Trailhead facilities
Lester-Amity Chalet has shelter, restrooms

Snow conditions
City of Duluth Parks & Rec hotline: 218-730-4321, press 1

What makes it unique
Lots of skiing on the edge of the city makes for a popular trail; the 6K of lighted trails are especially popular from dusk until late evening. The dramatic and majestic white pines along the lower loop by Amity Creek are a remnant of a forest that covered much of this area.

Information
City of Duluth Parks and Recreation, 218-730-4300. duluthmn.gov/parks/trails-bikeways/cross-country-ski-trails

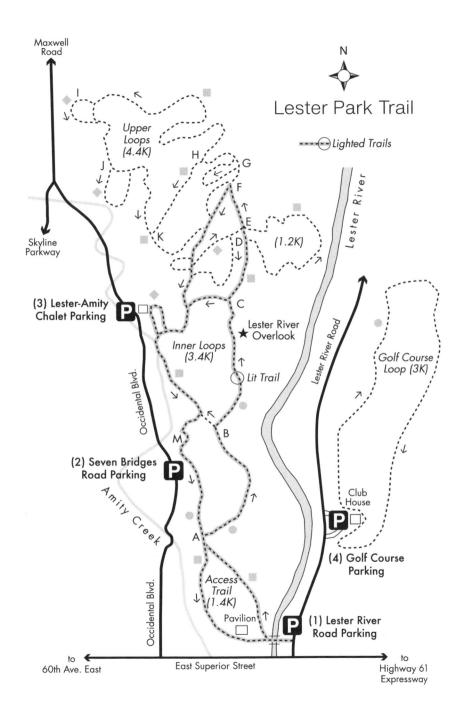

Maxwell
Road

N

Lester Park Trail

◉ *Lighted Trails*

I

*Upper
Loops
(4.4K)*

H   G

J   F

Skyline
Parkway   E

K   D   *(1.2K)*

Lester River

**(3) Lester-Amity
Chalet Parking**   P □

C

*Inner Loops
(3.4K)*   ★ Lester River
Overlook

Lester River Road

*Golf Course
Loop (3K)*

Occidental Blvd.

◉ *Lit Trail*

B

M

**(2) Seven Bridges
Road Parking**   P

Amity Creek

A

Club
House

P □

**(4) Golf Course
Parking**

Occidental Blvd.

*Access
Trail
(1.4K)*

Pavilion
□

P   **(1) Lester River
Road Parking**

to
60th Ave. East   East Superior Street

to
Highway 61
Expressway

ACCESS TRAIL (1.4K)

Intermediate/lighted. From the Lester River Road trailhead, cross the bridge, then climb through majestic white pine after crossing the open field. The first climb is pretty steep. On the return downhill run back into the open park field, you'll glide by huge pines and the scenic river—a real North Woods treat!

INNER LOOP (A-B-C) (3.4K)

Easier and more difficult/lighted. This is a very popular 3.4K loop which divides into: 1) an easier 2.0K southern loop that is one long, gradual climb and two gradual downhills; and 2) a 1.2K more difficult northern loop that is a little hillier. Many people start this loop from the lower Seven Bridges Road parking lot. Expect to share the trail with a mix of skier levels, from speedy skate skiers to leisurely families.

UPPER LOOPS (C-D-F-G-H-J-K) (4.4K PLUS SIDE LOOPS)

Intermediate and advanced/C-D-F lighted. This is really two trails. The main trail is 4.4K of intermediate skiing through mixed forest. It's a gradual climb into level terrain, followed by a bit of a roller coaster ride down. You'll get away from the crowds on this loop. You can add a quiet, relatively level 1.2K intermediate side loop on the way up.

The Upper Loops can also be an expert trail by adding the five advanced side loops, each about 0.5K. Each advanced side loop has both a steep climb and descent, not necessarily in that order. If you do all the side loops, this section ends up being around 9K. Caution: If you're not up for the hills and turns, watch out at intersections "I" and "J;" the intermediate trail goes left while the advanced trail goes straight ahead.

The Upper Loops, with their higher elevation, tend to have better snow conditions than are found on the lower loops.

GOLF COURSE LOOP (3K)

Easy/skijoring. The open, rolling terrain of the Lester Park Golf Course makes for a radically different skiing experience than the rest of Lester-Amity. This is not lighted, but is skiable at night by full moon (at your own risk). Grooming is a bit less frequent than the rest of the trails, but it's the only Duluth city park trail open to skijoring. You'll enjoy views of Lake Superior from the upper parts of the course. Park at the golf course clubhouse, 0.5 miles up Lester River Road from Superior Street.

LAKE SUPERIOR ICE IS NICE

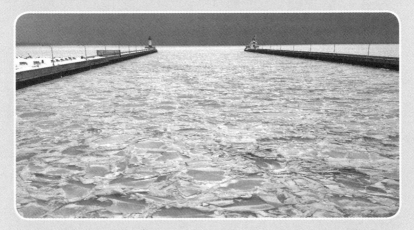

February and March are the best months for ice watchers. The water of Lake Superior is at its coldest in the month of March. Almost every year the shallower or more protected bays of the North Shore will freeze over during the late winter, but some years it is frozen as far as the eye can see. And once every twenty years or so, the whole lake freezes over—which takes a combination of a long-term cold winter, a serious cold snap, and relatively calm seas. This last happened during the years of 1978, 1994, and 2014. However, climate change experts predict we may never see a full freeze of Lake Superior again. ❄

Bagley Nature Area
Duluth, Minnesota

Trailhead access
Take St. Marie Street from Woodland Avenue to the Bagley Nature Area parking lot near Oakland Apartments.

Total groomed trail: 2.7K
Classic skiing: 2.7K

Trail difficulty
Bagley Nature Area offers fairly challenging trails for general usage. Real beginners should stick to the short-cut version of the East Loop.

Pass requirements
- None. Parking meters at trailhead are enforced 8am to 8pm, Monday through Friday.

Trailhead facilities
Outhouse

Snow conditions
Frequent reports on skinnyski.com

What makes it unique
A great asset for students is also available for community use. Bring a few quarters; you have to plug a meter for parking. Don't be surprised if walkers have been in the ski tracks before you.

Information
University of Minnesota Duluth Outdoor Program, (218) 726-6533. d.umn.edu/recreational-sports-outdoor-program/facilities/bagley-nature-center

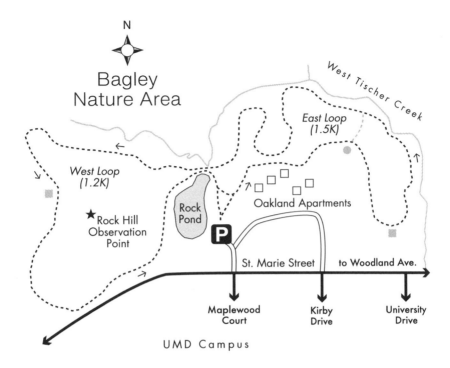

WEST LOOP (1.2K)

Intermediate. This is the more challenging of the two loops as you ski around Rock Hill, a former downhill ski area. The trail climbs for a long time through maple forest with some nice paper birch mixed in. Where the trail crosses a closed road to the top of Rock Hill, stop for some winter tree identification: there is maple, oak and basswood here—can you pick them out? A downhill run takes you back to Rock Pond.

EAST LOOP (1.5K)

Intermediate. Take a quick loop through UMD's maple sugarbush. This is mostly level terrain except for a steep section along Tischer Creek, where you will need to herringbone or sidestep. You can bypass this difficult section on a skier-groomed cutoff.

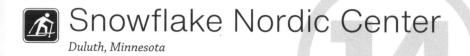

Snowflake Nordic Center
Duluth, Minnesota

Trailhead access
Take Rice Lake Road 0.5 mile north of Arrowhead Road. Entrance road is shared with tennis club.

Total groomed trail: 15K
Classic skiing: 15K   Skate skiing: 15K   Lighted trail: 6K

Pass requirements
• Day passes ($10) for sale at trailhead chalet. Season passes for sale online ($149 individual; $239 family; $89 student; generous early-bird discounts offered in November). All kids under age 5 ski free.

Trail difficulty
Snowflakde Nordic Center offers generally intermediate terrain, though trail builders took advantage of the landscape's few steep hills. The biggest challenge might be finding a parking spot on busy afternoons and weekends.

Trailhead facilities
Chalet with restrooms, changing rooms, sauna, and wax room. Rentals, kid and adult lessons, beverages, and snacks available. Hours: Monday-Saturday 8-8; Sunday 8-6.

Snow conditions
Frequent reports on skinnyski.com

What makes it unique
Thanks to the boundless energy of the legendary George Hovland (who was on the 1952 Oslo Olympics ski team), Snowflake Nordic Center provides high-quality grooming and facilities right in town. When conditions are marginal, your best bet for good skiing in Duluth is here. Snowflake is frequented by ski racers and hosts local high school and college ski teams for practices as well as races. Sundays can get busy with kid ski programs, skijoring races, and more.

Information
Snowflake Nordic Center, 218 726-1550, skiduluth.com

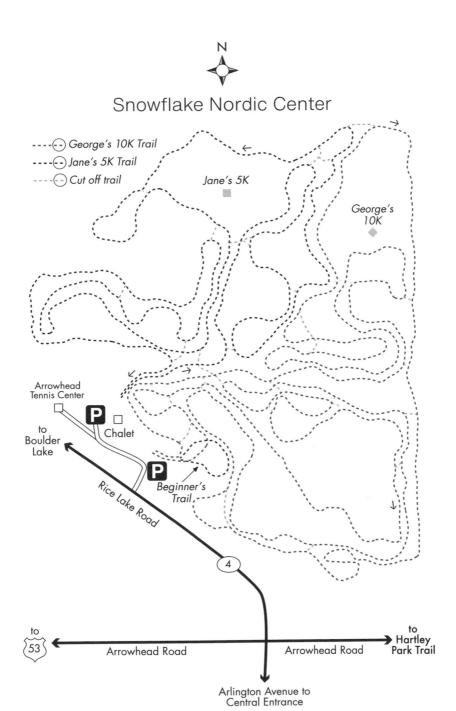

Snowflake Nordic Center

--- ⊙ George's 10K Trail
--- ⊙ Jane's 5K Trail
--- ⊙ Cut off trail

Jane's 5K

George's
10K

Arrowhead
Tennis Center

to
Boulder
Lake

P Chalet

P

Beginner's
Trail

Rice Lake Road

4

to
53

Arrowhead Road

Arrowhead Road

to
Hartley
Park Trail

Arlington Avenue to
Central Entrance

JANE'S 5K (5K)

Intermediate/lighted. This loop is trickiest at the start and finish, with short, steep climbs to challenge any skier. However, the middle "half" is relatively flat, with the main challenge coming from tight curves—this is a nice stretch to focus on technique. The lighting is effective if a little unromantic, with power lines strung from tree to tree. Ignore the other lights and trails and settle in for the curvy "here and now."

GEORGE'S 10K (10K)

Advanced. If you're strictly into getting from Point A to Point B, this trail is not for you and might, in fact, drive you a bit crazy. But if you're into the aesthetics of a well-groomed trail and a well-designed curve, be sure to check this trail out; don't even try to keep your bearings here. This loop squeezes a great variety of terrain out of a tight area, beginning with some steep ups and downs. If the first hills intimidated you, hold on; you've made it through the only truly advanced stretch of the loop. The rest is classic intermediate terrain and leads into birch and evergreen forest. Various cutoffs let you shorten the overall distance, if desired.

COME NORTH, SKI LOVERS

Compared to the Twin Cities, the North Shore is skiers' heaven. Sure, an early storm might go south and bring city-dwellers a few days of great skiing. But week after week, the most reliable snow and skiing conditions in Minnesota are on the Shore. Duluth has 109 days per winter with at least six inches of snow, and Grand Marais has 94; Minneapolis has just 54. Around the Flathorn-Gegoka trails, there's over 90 days a year with snow over 12 inches deep; Saint Paul averages 20 days a year with snow like that. Every five miles north on I-35 brings an additional inch of average snow per year. ❄

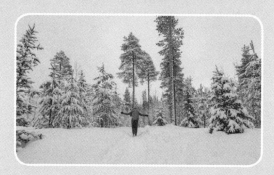

Boulder Lake Ski Trail
Duluth, Minnesota

Trailhead access
Boulder Lake is 18 miles north of Duluth. Take Highway 4 north past Island Lake, then turn left on Boulder Dam Road. There are four trailheads along Boulder Dam Road: **(1)** The large and popular **Bear Paw trailhead,** with its intermediate trails; **(2)** The smaller and quieter **Rolling Pin trailhead** by Nordberg Road, with advanced trails; **(3)** The smallest and quietest **Boat Launch trailhead** at Boulder Dam at the end of the road, with the easy Otter Run trail; **(4)** and the **East trailhead,** just off of Boulder Dam Road and Boulder Lake Road, with access to easy, longer loops. All trails in this system are connected.

Total groomed trail: 19.2K
Classic skiing: 19.2K   Skate skiing: 11K

Trail difficulty
Each trailhead (see above) provides a different degree of difficulty access.

Pass requirements
• None

Trailhead facilities
Outhouses at most trailheads. Wolfski's Ski Den warming shack has hot beverages, and is open dawn to dusk.

Snow conditions
Skier's hotline 218-721-4903, facebook.com/BoulderLakeELC

What makes it unique
The trails are built on land owned by Minnesota Power, St. Louis County, and the state near the shores of lovely Boulder Lake. Skiers can rest and snack at the warming cabin, ski across frozen Boulder Lake, and connect to a wide array of trails on the other side. With so many trailhead options, it's also easy to jump directly onto your favorite trails in the system.

Information
Boulder Lake Environmental Center, blma.org

ROLLING PIN/RIDGE RUNNER/TIMBER CRUISER (2.4K)

Intermediate to expert/classic only. These three trails form a figure eight using a glacial esker for the "cross." Because of the one-way markings, most skiers will ski all three. Rolling Pin winds you around to the start of Ridge Runner, which traces the top of an esker. Timber Cruiser starts with a steep downhill coming off of the esker and runs through a recently logged area.

OTTER RUN (2.4K)

Beginner/classic only. This curvy loop trail is the easiest part of the system; with its own trailhead, it's perfect for a beginner. The forest is incredibly diverse here, with mature white pine at the western end, plus maple, large-toothed aspen, and ash. The trail is level and easy going. Beginners will want to access this loop from the Boat Launch trailhead (#3) to avoid the hills at the Rolling Pin trailhead.

BEAR PAW (2.3K)

Intermediate/skating and classic. Access this trail either from the Bear Paw or Rolling Pin trailheads—the latter trailhead by heading across Boulder Lake itself at the warming hut, on a trail across the frozen lake (follow the trees stuck in the snow). This loop takes you through a young aspen forest with occasional patches of old white pine. A few easy hills make this barely an intermediate trail.

BLUE OX (3.8K)

Intermediate/skating and classic. Babe the Blue Ox was Paul Bunyan's helper in logging the mighty pines. This trail shows the "before" and "after" of Babe's work. The first half of this loop rolls gently through a white pine forest that survived a major blow down in 2016. The second half of the loop takes you through vigorous regrowth of aspen and birch. It's a good place to take an advanced beginner for his or her first big loop.

NINE PINE (4.7K)

Intermediate/skating and classic. If you enjoyed Blue Ox, cross the snowmobile trail and experience very similar terrain, with a few additional thrills and spills. The "Can of Nerves" takes you through a steep hairpin in a dark piney forest.

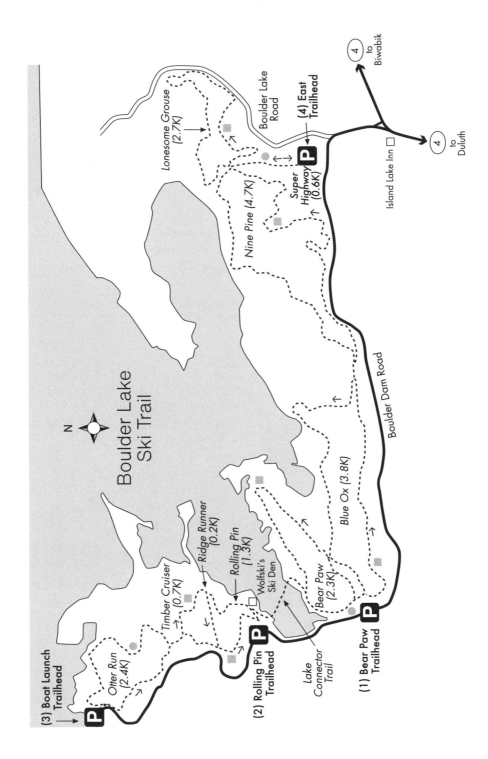

Boulder Lake Ski Trail

N

to Biwabik

to Duluth

Island Lake Inn

(4) East Trailhead

Boulder Lake Road

Lonesome Grouse (2.7K)

Super Highway (0.6K)

Nine Pine (4.7K)

Boulder Dam Road

Blue Ox (3.8K)

Bear Paw (2.3K)

Ridge Runner (0.2K)

Rolling Pin (1.3K)

Wolfski's Ski Den

Timber Cruiser (0.7K)

Otter Run (2.4K)

(3) Boat Launch Trailhead

(2) Rolling Pin Trailhead

Lake Connector Trail

(1) Bear Paw Trailhead

LONESOME GROUSE (2.7K)

Intermediate/classic only. While marked on maps as an "intermediate" trail, this is actually a pleasant beginner trail through intimate aspen and fir forest. Double-tracked, this is a perfect trail for skiing and chatting with a friend. You can make an easy day of skiing by parking at the East trailhead (#4), heading out on the Super Highway, and completing this trail for a 3.8K total outing.

SUPER HIGHWAY (0.6K)

Beginner/skating and classic. You'll find a wide-open trail here with double classic tracks on both sides. The trail is mostly used by skiers who park at the East trailhead and access Lonesome Grouse and Ninepine trails.

TRACKING BACKWARDS

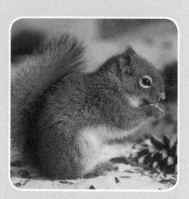

Animals such as the red squirrel, snowshoe hare, and deer mouse are hoppers, and their tracks show an unusual pattern. After an animal hops, it lands first on its front feet. Then its back feet come down in front of the front feet. The snowshoe hare track is found near areas with thick underbrush; the much smaller red squirrel track generally runs from tree to tree in coniferous forests. You can always tell which way a hopper was headed; just think backwards. ❄

Biskey Ponds Ski Trail

Fredenberg Township, Minnesota

Trailhead access
Drive north from Duluth on Lavaque Road (County Road 48). Turn left (on Fish Lake Road) by the well-known Fredenberg "Minno-ette" convenience store. Follow Fish Lake Road for 0.9 miles, then turn left on Fish Lake Dam Rd. Follow Fish Lake Dam Road for 2.2 miles. Trailhead parking lot on the right. Recommend using smart phone to navigate to "Biskey Ponds Nordic Ski Trail".

Total groomed trail: 12K
Classic skiing: 12K

Trail difficulty
Intimate and narrow classic trails are fun and keep your attention. The Wolf Run corridor and the Black Spruce trail are both level to gently rolling terrain. Loops on the western side are more challenging, with some short and steep hills.

Pass requirements
• None. Donation box at trailhead.

Trailhead facilities
None

Snow conditions
biskeypondsnordic.wordpress.com

What makes it unique
One of the newer trails in the Duluth area is as old-fashioned as it gets, with handmade wooden signs, narrow, classic-only trails, and regular grooming by the Fredenberg Flyers Ski Club. The hardest part is finding the trailhead; it's an indirect, winding, 30-40 minute drive north of Duluth. Though there's been significant forest management on these County lands, it feels wild and remote here.

Information
biskeypondsnordic.wordpress.com

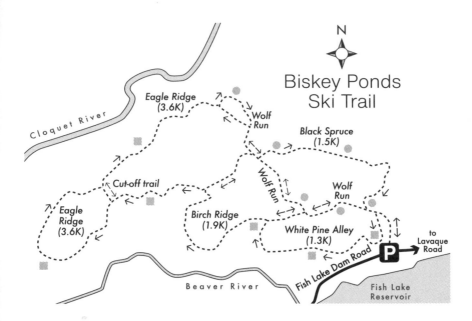

Biskey Ponds
Ski Trail

Eagle Ridge
(3.6K)

Cloquet River

Wolf
Run

Black Spruce
(1.5K)

Cut-off trail

Wolf Run

Wolf
Run

Eagle
Ridge
(3.6K)

Birch Ridge
(1.9K)

White Pine Alley
(1.3K)

to
Lavaque
Road

Fish Lake Dam Road

Beaver River

Fish Lake
Reservoir

WOLF RUN (2K)

Easy. This main corridor trail follows an old road and is double-tracked. All other loops on this system start and end on Wolf Run, so you'll see frequent single-track trails spinning off into the woods. Just before the far northern end, there's a short "lollipop" of less than 1K. If you're looking for a beginner's outing, this is a perfect trail—it's 4K out and back.

BLACK SPRUCE (1.5K)

Easy. This newer trail gives you the option of a 2.5K beginner loop when you take Wolf Run nearly to its end and then turn right onto Black Spruce. The trail runs gently downhill into a lovely black spruce swamp, where you'll find interesting bog vegetation like Labrador tea popping out of the snow.

WHITE PINE ALLEY (1.3K)

Intermediate. This is the first loop off to left side of Wolf Run. The single-tracked trail leads past numerous ponds and past big pines. For a long ski, use White Pine Alley to start a 8.5K tour of the entire outside perimeter of this trail system, taking all the one-ways on White Pine Alley, Birch Ridge and Eagle Ridge, and finishing with Black Spruce.

BIRCH RIDGE (1.9K)

Intermediate. The trail climbs through paper birch and poplar trees, which look beautiful on a blue-sky, winter day. The Beaver River, to the south, flows from Fish Lake into the Cloquet River. The Fredenberg Flyers Ski Club calls the hills here "moderate but exciting!"

EAGLE RIDGE (3.6K)

Intermediate. Although ranked intermediate, this is the most challenging stretch of trail in the system, with steep climbs and downhill glides. It also has the best views and an amazing stretch of beautiful conifer trees, including groves of tall white pines. The two-way cut-off trail lets you skip the big hill...or ski it again.

RESOURCES FOR SKIERS

The North Shore is a full-service skiing destination with cross-country ski equipment rentals, restaurants, and lodging—from remote, rustic cabins to elegant urban hotels—found along the way.

North Shore Chambers and Associations
- Visit Duluth, visitduluth.com
- Lake County Chamber of Commerce, lakecounty-chamber.com
- Visit Cook County, visitcookcounty.com

Ski Conditions
- skinnyski.com — skier-posted reports from around the region
- City of Duluth ski trail conditions: 218-730-4321
- Department of Natural Resources snow depth and groomed trail conditions, dnr.state.mn.us/snow_depth/index.html

Ski Rentals and Equipment
- Hartley Nature Center, Duluth MN, 218-724-6735
- UMD Outdoor Program (near Bagley Nature Area), 218-726-6134
- Continental Ski & Bike, Duluth MN 218-728-4466
- Ski Hut, Duluth MN, 218-724-8525, theskihut.com
- Snowflake Nordic, Duluth MN, skiduluth.com
- Sawtooth Outfitters, Tofte MN, 218-663-7643, sawtoothoutfitters. com (direct access to the Sugarbush Trail System)
- Devils Track Nordic Ski Shop, Grand Marais MN, 218-387-3373, devilstracknordic.com (direct access to Pincushion Mountain)

Road Conditions
- Minnesota: 511mn.org
- Wisconsin: 511wi.gov

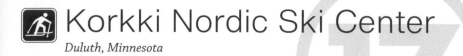

Korkki Nordic Ski Center

Duluth, Minnesota

Trailhead access
Take Homestead Road (County Road 42) 2.5 miles north from milepost 14.9 on Highway 61 expressway, to left turn at Korkki Road. Go west on Korkki Road (County Road 43) for 0.5 miles to Nordic Center entrance on right.

Total groomed trail: 11K
Classic skiing: 11K

Trail difficulty
Most skiers will find that Korkki Nordic offers challenging terrain, but the hills and curves are so well laid out you'll feel more thrilled than scared.

Pass requirements
- None. Donation box at trailhead (suggested donation $3–$5). Korkki Nordic Ski Center was formed as a nonprofit organization dedicated to maintaining traditional Nordic skiing at this premiere trail system. Annual memberships encouraged.

Trailhead facilities
Chalet with wood stove and changing room. Outhouse.

Snow conditions
Frequent reports on skinnyski.com

What makes it unique
These are truly "Charlie's Trails," as they are affectionately called by those in the know. Charlie Banks was one of the legendary figures of Duluth skiing, and built these trails himself in 1955 on public land in his "backyard." The club maintains the trail and its history and character, preserving traditional single-track, classic skiing and a sense of community. Korkki Nordic has been called "possibly the prettiest trail on the North Shore."

Information
You'll find interesting trail history and fun background information on the many trail signs online at korkkinordic.org.

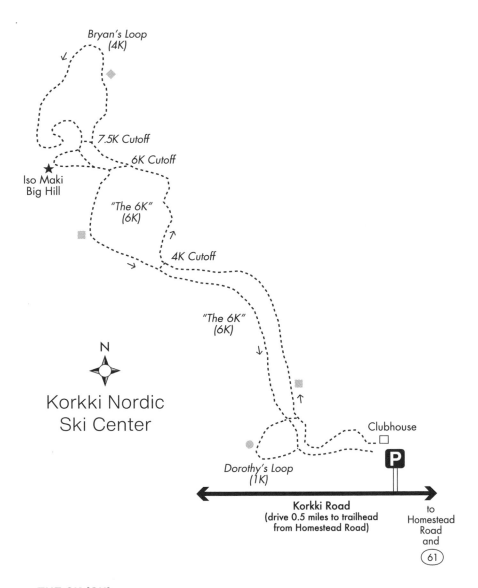

Bryan's Loop
(4K)

7.5K Cutoff

6K Cutoff

Iso Maki
Big Hill

"The 6K"
(6K)

4K Cutoff

"The 6K"
(6K)

N

Korkki Nordic
Ski Center

Clubhouse

P

Dorothy's Loop
(1K)

Korkki Road
(drive 0.5 miles to trailhead
from Homestead Road)

to
Homestead
Road
and
(61)

THE 6K (6K)

Intermediate. This is single-tracked and narrow, with exciting hills where you can't see the bottom and where you'll throw caution to the wind... but it all works out fine. You gradually climb through mixed forest and ash swamps, then return on a gradual and wonderful downhill run that makes you feel like a champion skier. There are two especially challenging parts of the downhill run, when the trail goes down and back up along a river bank. Most skiers stay on the main trail through these features, and beginning skiers can avoid these more difficult sections by taking the easier side trails.

BRYAN'S LOOP (4K)

Advanced. Skiers choosing the "whole enchilada" will experience more challenging terrain, with some sharp turns on steep hills. There are beaver ponds and piney ridges (known as "Wolf Kill Ridge") back here, too. The middle third of the loop is relatively level and in open woods, but the last third has a hairpin turn and other thrills. The "Iso Maki Big Hill," also available to those who take the 7.5K cutoff, is a steep climb to a great view from the top of inland ridges, and a speedy run down a hill that seems to go on forever. A cutoff is available to those who want to skip the big downhill.

DOROTHY'S LOOP (1K)

Easier. Apparently Charlie Banks' wife Dorothy did not like skiing on hills. Flatter and wider than the main loop, this is perfect for beginners, kids, and instructional outings—you just have to take the first swooping hill on the system to get here. True beginners should ski the loop clockwise.

KORKKI NORDIC SKI CENTER

Your donation to Korkki helps maintain traditional Nordic skiing on this spectacular trail. Annual membership is $30 for families and $20 for individuals. For memberships visit **korkkinordic.org** or use the donation box at trailhead.

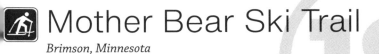

Mother Bear Ski Trail

Brimson, Minnesota

Trailhead access
On St. Louis County Road 44, 2 miles southwest of Brimson and 9 miles northeast of Pequaywan Lakes (about 35 miles from eastern Duluth, or about a 1-hour drive). From Korkki Nordic and Highway 61, it's a fun and winding 40-minute drive along county roads 42, 41, and 266 to 44.

Total groomed trail: 10.7 K
Classic skiing: 10.7K

Trail difficulty
Stay in the first set of loops and it's pretty easy terrain here. Out on the remote western loops, the trail gets trickier and fewer people ski here, so be extra careful.

Pass requirements
• Great Minnesota Ski Pass

Trailhead facilities
Outhouse

Snow conditions
facebook.com/motherbearskitrail

What makes it unique
Off the beaten path, this trail primarily serves local residents. Because this trail is not used as often as others, and because the forest is so varied here, the animal tracking can be superb. Watch for signs of wolf, lynx, and snowshoe hare, especially on the South Loop.

Information
facebook.com/motherbearskitrail

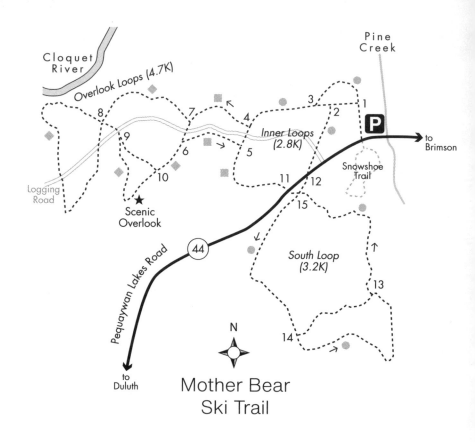

Mother Bear
Ski Trail

INNER LOOPS (2.8K)

Easy to difficult. These are intersections marked 1-5. From marker 1 counterclockwise around past 2 and 3 to 4, it's a gradual run through a variety of conifers and then an open area. Beginners should turn around at marker 4 and retrace their tracks, as the trail to marker 15 takes some steep downhill turns without much room to snowplow.

SOUTH LOOP (3.2K)

Easy. A longer, gentle loop through beautiful pine forest, with a more challenging side trail from 14 to 13. You have to cross the highway to get to these trails, but it's worth the effort.

OVERLOOK LOOPS (4.7K)

Expert. This is a series of loops with scenic views, crisscrossing a logging road. Most of the loops are one-way counterclockwise. You can take just one or do all three. The 4-7-6-5 loop starts with a big climb through young aspen and ends with a fun, tricky downhill. Only adventurous skiers should attempt the curvy, skier-groomed trail from 7 to 8. The 6-10-9 loop runs through a boggy area and on top of what appears to be a glacial esker. The last 1.6K loop starts and ends at 8 and leads to an overlook of the Cloquet River and the edge of a rim overlooking a spruce bog below.

TRACKS OF THE LONG AND LEAN

The North Woods have many long and lean members of the weasel family, and they all leave a distinctive track pattern, a pair of prints nearly side by side but slightly offset. Each set of tracks is between one and three feet away from the next, representing the "bound" of the sinuous animals. This is actually a running gait, with the front feet landing first and the rear feet landing exactly in the prints left by the front feet.

The two most common weasels leaving tracks by ski trails are the pine marten and the fisher. The two animals are similar enough in size that their tracks are hard to tell apart; a smaller footprint (just less than two inches long) would be a marten and a larger set (just slightly more than two inches long) would be a fisher, but there's lots of room in between. Use habitat as a clue: marten are found in the mature boreal forest where they can chase squirrels through the trees. The fisher often captures porcupine and prefers a more open successional forest. ❄

Lake County

State parks and local volunteers. Skiing in Lake County gives you a new appreciation for both. The North Shore state parks stand out on maps, from the diverse trail network at Gooseberry Falls State Park to the deep woods and dramatic terrain of Tettegouche State Park. You'll also find some gems tucked into the hills, like Silver Bay's Northwoods Ski Touring Trail and Two Harbors' Erkki Harju Ski Trail, both maintained by local volunteers. Away from the shore and on the edge of the Boundary Waters Canoe Area Wilderness, explore deep snow and towering pines at the Flathorn-Gegoka Ski Trail. Given the bounty of cross-country skiing here, maybe they should change the name of Lake County to "Snow County!"

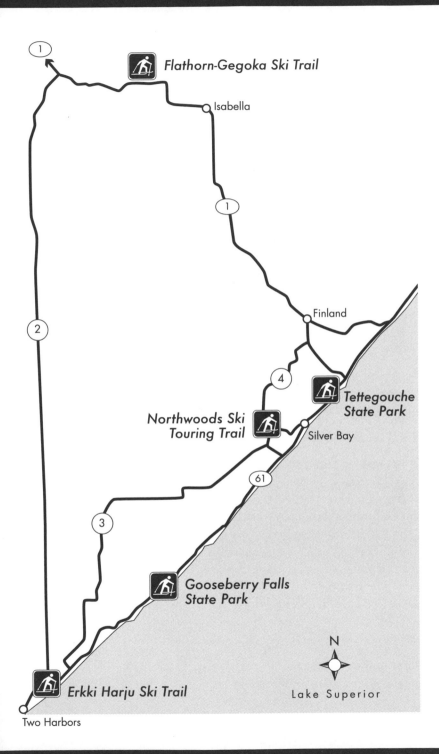

Flathorn-Gegoka Ski Trail

Isabella

Finland

Tettegouche
State Park

Northwoods Ski
Touring Trail

Silver Bay

Gooseberry Falls
State Park

Erkki Harju Ski Trail

Two Harbors

N

Lake Superior

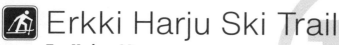

Erkki Harju Ski Trail

Two Harbors, Minnesota

Trailhead access
Take County Road 2 from Highway 61 north 0.7 miles until signed entrance to parking lot on the right side of the road.

Total groomed trail: 9K
Classic skiing: 9K   Skate skiing: 9K

Trail difficulty
Erkki Harju offers primarily easier trails, but a few optional side loops add spice to your skiing.

Pass requirements
• Great Minnesota Ski Pass
• Membership in Two Harbors Ski Club encouraged

Trailhead facilities
None

Snow Conditions
facebook.com/2harborsskitrail

What makes it unique
This is a gentle, quiet system of ski trails well used and loved by local families and the high school ski team. The 3K inside loop is the only lighted trail between Duluth and Grand Marais. Erkki was a Two Harbors carpenter and ski enthusiast who immigrated from Finland in 1956. He was the first person ever to ski 100 kilometers in a single day on the Korkki Nordic trails.

Information
facebook.com/2harborsskitrail

> ## ERKKI HARJU SKI TRAIL
>
> Support the locals who maintain this community trail. Membership in the Two Harbors Ski Club is $10 for individuals; $15 for families. Send your checks to Two Harbors Ski Trail, PO Box 381, Two Harbors MN, 55616.

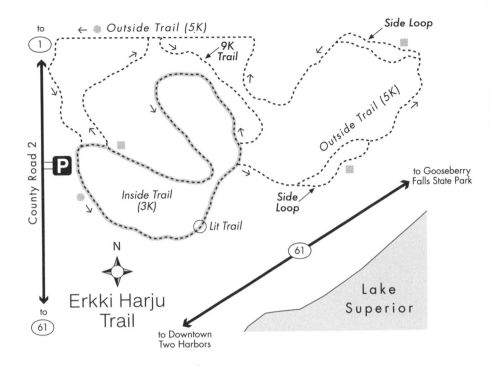

INSIDE TRAIL (3K)

Intermediate/lighted. This inside loop forms the outline of a "C" as it runs through the strips of forest between the fairways of Lakeview National Golf Course. The open fairways provide an airy feel to your ski. The trail lights look like little lighthouses along the way and are actually airstrip runway lights.

OUTSIDE TRAIL (5K, PLUS 1K ADVANCED SIDE LOOPS)

Easier to advanced. The terrain is gently rolling, with few uphills or downhills. This trail leaves the golf course fairways behind. Two side loops of about 0.5K each are for advanced skiers, with quick turns and sharp climbs. Toward the end of the loop, once you have your bearings, you can weave between the 3K and the 5K loops for a total 9K ski outing.

Gooseberry Falls State Park

Two Harbors, Minnesota

Trailhead access
Take Visitor Center/Wayside Rest exit off Highway 61, twelve miles northeast of Two Harbors. Go either to Visitor Center or to Lakeview picnic shelter on lakeshore.

Total groomed trail: 20K
Classic skiing: 20K   Skate skiing: 5K

Trail difficulty
If the snow is good, beginners can stay on the Highway 61 lake side of the park. Getting to the vast network of the park's inland trails is trickier, but highly rewarding—intermediate skiers will find long loops and beautiful terrain.

Pass Requirements
- Great Minnesota Ski Pass (self-service permits available at park)
- Minnesota State Parks vehicle permit (required only when using the Lakeview Picnic Center trailhead)

Trailhead facilities
Restrooms, snacks, warming room, gift shop, and visitor center.

Snow conditions
dnr.state.mn.us/snow_depth/trails.html?facility_id=4128

What makes it unique
Gooseberry Falls State Park is the first large trail system as you head up the North Shore. Its diverse terrain and remote trails make it a favorite for a full day of skiing. Families with young children can use the beautiful lobby of the visitor center as a warming hut—and parents can take turns exploring the trails.

Information
Gooseberry Falls State Park, 218-595-7100, dnr.state.mn.us/parkfinder/index.html

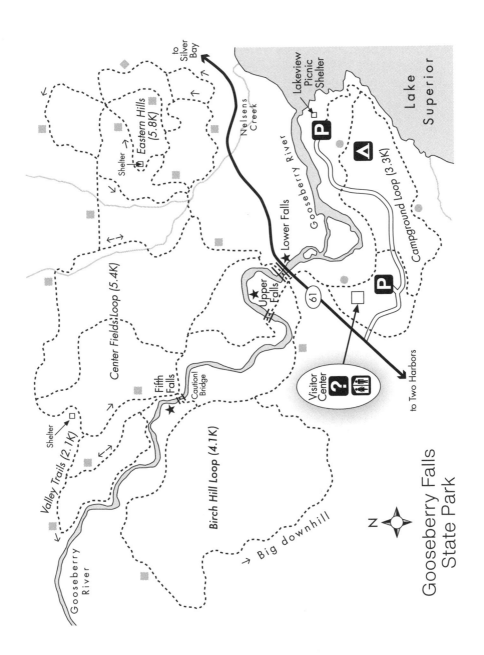

Gooseberry Falls
State Park

N

to Silver Bay

Lakeview
Picnic
Shelter

Lake
Superior

Shelter →

Eastern Hills
(5.8K)

Nelsens Creek

Gooseberry River

Lower Falls

Campground Loop (3.3K)

Center Fields Loop (5.4K)

Upper
Falls

61

to Two Harbors

Fifth
Falls

Caution!
Bridge

Shelter

Valley Trails (2.1K)

Visitor
Center

Birch Hill Loop (4.1K)

→ Big downhill

Gooseberry River

CAMPGROUND LOOP (3.3K)

Easy. Take this trail either direction through the open woods of the lakeshore and campground area. You can start from the Visitor Center area, or if you have a vehicle permit you can start on the 0.3K spur from Lakeview picnic shelter by Agate Beach. The views to the Gooseberry River valley and the icy Lake Superior shoreline are among the most dramatic of all North Shore trails. The trail crosses a park road twice, so you may have to take off your skis or step gingerly across the pavement.

Inland trails

Access these trails from the Visitor Center. A busy, main feeder trail parallels a snowmobile trail underneath the highway bridge on the west side of river, with a dramatic view of the Upper Falls.

BIRCH HILL LOOP (4.1K)

More difficult/classic and skating. After crossing under Highway 61, you will take a 0.7K access trail to this remote loop. Watch for the deer exclosure just past the junction with the trail down to Fifth Falls. After a steep climb to the open ridgeline, get ready for a fun, gradual 1.2K downhill run. When you finally have to kick again, it will be in a pleasant, open forest. Use caution as you near the highway, as the trail is shared with snowmobiles and the last turn down to the bridge is tricky.

CENTER FIELDS LOOP (5.4K)

More difficult. Cross the pedestrian bridge which runs over the Gooseberry River and under the highway. Or head up the Birch Hill loop and cross the river on a snowmobile bridge. This is open country of spruce and birch. The main counterclockwise loop is 4.4K of trail from the bridge. It's great for relaxed cruising, especially on a sunny day when you can stop at the shelter and bask in the rays. Take off from this main loop onto either of the sections below for a full adventure. Enjoy a break at the Fifth Falls bridge, or use the bridge to reach the Birch Hill Loop, but do take off your skis before heading downhill to the bridge.

VALLEY TRAILS (2.1K)

More difficult. If the skiing is fast, this section can be scary and should be rated most difficult. Downhill runs come off the Center Fields loop and scoot you down to the banks of the Gooseberry River, where you will cruise past huge cedar trees. The climb back up the river bank is fairly long and steep.

EASTERN HILLS (5.8K)

More difficult to most difficult. Head out into this section, and if you are comfortable with some hills and turns, forget about the trail maps that show up every few hundred meters and just follow your curiosity up and down and around these hills. You won't get lost, but you will enjoy open country of birch and spruce forest. One 0.8K section is rated advanced for its tight turns and sharp hills; it also connects with an ungroomed trail to a neighboring lodge. If you make it to the shelter, pull out a snack and enjoy the view!

WARMER BY THE LAKE

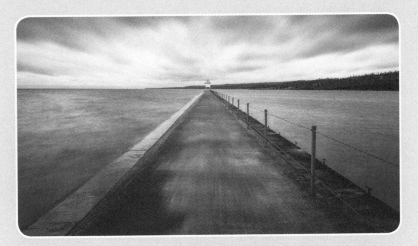

Some call the North Shore the "Norwegian Riviera." Believe it or not, North Shore communities can be the warmest places in Minnesota when it's really cold statewide. Lake Superior water has an average temperature of 39 degrees Fahrenheit. In summer, the lake acts like a big ice cube and keeps us cool; in winter, it acts like a big radiator and keeps us warm. ❄

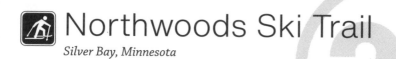

Northwoods Ski Trail

Silver Bay, Minnesota

Trailhead access
Take Outer Drive, which becomes Penn Boulevard and Superior National Forest Scenic Byway, through the town of Silver Bay for a total of 3.2 miles from Highway 61 (past a parking area for the Superior Hiking Trail) to signed parking area on right.

Total groomed trail: 19K
Classic skiing: 19K

Trail difficulty
With narrow, classic trails—and hills found on every loop—this is not a trail system for true beginners.

Pass Requirements
• Great Minnesota Ski Pass
• Use donation box at trailhead to support this trail system groomed by volunteers.

Trailhead facilities
None

Snow conditions
Check skinnyski.com trail reports for skier updates

What makes it unique
This local trail adds a traditional twist to North Shore skiing. The narrow trails and great views make this feel like you are on the Superior Hiking Trail. Bean Lake is a favorite destination for hikers in the summer on the SHT, and for skiers in the winter on this trail.

Information
Northwoods Ski Touring Club, 218-226-4334

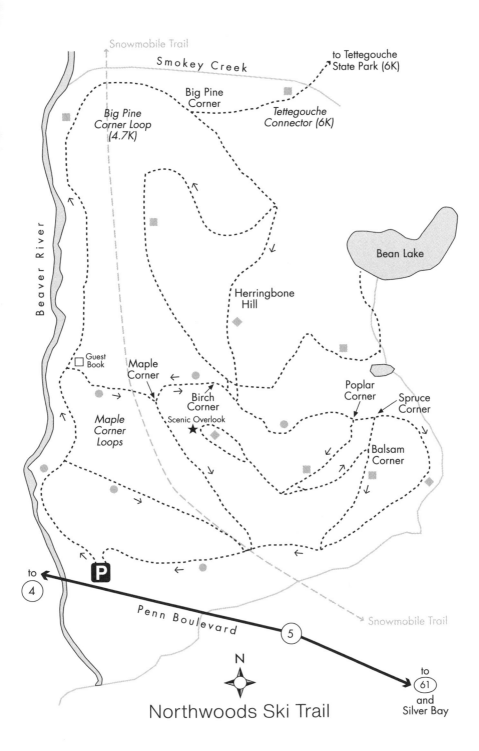

Snowmobile Trail

Smokey Creek

to Tettegouche
State Park (6K)

Big Pine
Corner

Big Pine
Corner Loop
(4.7K)

Tettegouche
Connector (6K)

Beaver River

Bean Lake

Herringbone
Hill

Guest
Book

Maple
Corner

Birch
Corner

Poplar
Corner

Spruce
Corner

Scenic Overlook

Maple
Corner
Loops

Balsam
Corner

to
4

P

Penn Boulevard

5

Snowmobile Trail

to
61
and
Silver Bay

N

Northwoods Ski Trail

MAPLE CORNER LOOPS (4.4K)

Easier. These beginner loops quickly immerse you in the intimacy of this trail system as you climb along the banks of the east branch of the Beaver River. Be sure to sign in at the trail register...and check out the colorful comments of your fellow skiers. It's 2.8K around the outside loop and 2.1K around the inside loop. Use caution on the two snowmobile trail crossings. There are fun and easy downhill runs with mountain-like views.

BIG PINE CORNER LOOP (4.7K)

Intermediate to advanced. This trail weaves up and into the open country of the Beaver River and its tributary, Smokey Creek, to Big Pine Corner, crisscrossing a snowmobile trail then turning south. From there you can either huff it over Herringbone Hill, 0.9K of a big up and down, or turn right onto a more level trail. Either way, the inland scenery is dramatic.

POPLAR/SPRUCE/BALSAM CORNERS (3.9K)

Intermediate to advanced. The side trails and scenic loop are for advanced skiers. Either climb up from Poplar Corner to the panoramic scenic overlook or descend from Spruce Corner into the rolling hillside. The downhill runs are particularly challenging here: be prepared for a strategic wipe-out, if necessary.

BEAN LAKE SPUR (1.1K)

Intermediate. Ski in from the major intersection of Birch Corner and past a large beaver pond into the rugged territory of Bean Lake. Three different trails converge at the same place on the lake, so be careful on your way back that you choose the right one.

TETTEGOUCHE CONNECTOR (6K)

Intermediate. Because of the distance involved and the remoteness, this section should only be skied by experienced, prepared skiers. But if you're prepared and conditions are favorable, this trail is a don't-miss experience. After crossing Smokey Creek, the trail follows the creek's upper reaches in a valley which gets narrower and narrower until you pass through a gorge with 250-foot cliffsides. The last few kilometers before Tettegouche Camp are on state park hiking trails and are difficult to groom well, so they might feel more rugged. The Connector trail eventually links with Tettegouche State Park. See the Tettegouche State Park section for a description of that trailhead and its trails. Perhaps your group has two cars and if so, this is an ideal A to B trail experience, with a car shuttle return to where you began.

SPLIT ROCK LIGHTHOUSE STATE PARK

Split Rock Lighthouse, that lonely sentinel atop a steep Lake Superior cliff, is a well-known Minnesota icon. Less well known is Split Rock Lighthouse State Park, which completely surrounds the lighthouse. Winter explorers will find a bit of everything to explore and enjoy in this park.

Many of the trails here used to be groomed for cross-country skiing. Park managers eventually realized that the trails were too winding and hilly for skiing; today they are perfect for snowshoeing and fat biking.

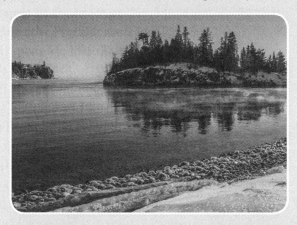

Start your adventure at the park's trail center, where you'll find warm indoor spaces and restrooms with running water. Trails leave right from the front door.

Snowshoers have the run of the park. Head out on the wider, groomed trails, then venture out on side trails to gorgeous overlooks like Corundum Point or Day Hill. You can rent snowshoes at the State Park visitor center.

Fat bikers have eight miles of trails. There's a 4-mile loop to the mouth of the Split Rock River, or cross Highway 61 and explore the upper park, including a long run along the old Merrill Logging Railroad. You can rent fat bikes at SpokeNGear in Two Harbors.

Be sure to check out the park's rugged coves and beaches. If you're lucky... and careful...you might be able to explore the shoreline ice.

The cart-in campground has sites that are open all winter, so Split Rock Lighthouse State Park could be your weekend destination for winter fun. ❋

Tettegouche State Park

Silver Bay, Minnesota

Trailhead access
Take Highway 61 four miles northeast of Silver Bay to park entrance. With a state park vehicle permit, head up the park access road 1.5 miles to parking lot at trailhead.

Total groomed trail: 13.5K
Classic skiing: 13.5K   Skate skiing: 7.5K

Trail difficulty
Every trail here has some sort of wild and fast downhill, but trails are groomed wide enough to keep it safe should you need to snowplow or take a fall.

Pass requirements
• Great Minnesota Ski Pass
• Minnesota State Parks vehicle permit

Trailhead facilities
Outhouses

Snow conditions
dnr.state.mn.us/snow_depth/ trails.html?facility_id=4193

What makes it unique
Long loops into quiet, dramatic country make for a real sense of adventure. The restored log cabins of Tettegouche Camp provide a unique ski-in overnight adventure deep inside the park.

Information
Tettegouche State Park
218-226-6365
dnr.state.mn.us/parkfinder/index.html

TETTEGOUCHE CAMP CABINS
Tettegouche State Park offers rustic, ski-in only lodging in four log cabins at Tettegouche Camp. The cabins sit on the shoreline of Mic Mac Lake in the middle of this trail system. Reservations are available up to 120 days in advance; complete details are on the park's webpage.

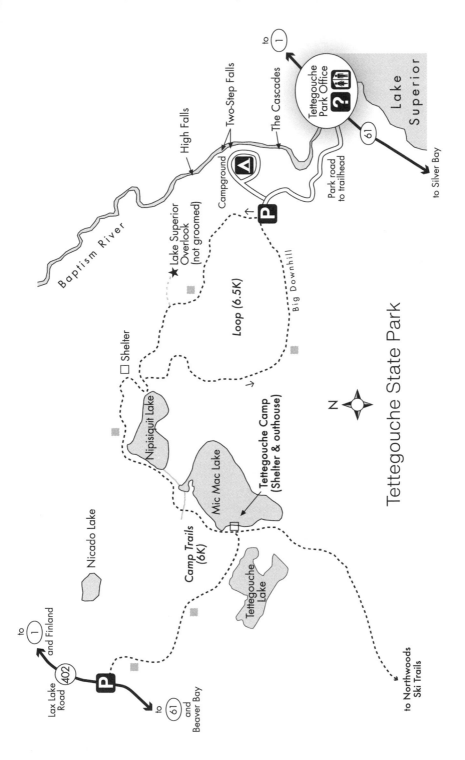

Tettegouche State Park

Baptism River

High Falls
Two-Step Falls
The Cascades

Tettegouche Park Office

Lake Superior

to 1

to Silver Bay

61

Park road to trailhead

Campground

★ Lake Superior Overlook (not groomed)

Loop (6.5K)

Big Downhill

Shelter

Nipisiquit Lake

Mic Mac Lake

Tettegouche Camp (Shelter & outhouse)

N

Nicado Lake

Camp Trails (6K)

Tettegouche Lake

to Northwoods Ski Trails

Lax Lake Road 402

to 1 and Finland

P

to 61 and Beaver Bay

LOOP TRAIL (6.5K)

Intermediate/skating and classic. This is a quintessential North Shore ski outing, where you will climb through a variety of habitats, then enjoy a thrilling downhill run back to the trailhead. Throw into the mix a lovely inland lake, majestic trees, and almost 5K of skiing without an intersection to worry about. The 2.9K climb to Nipisiquit Lake is nice enough, with a mix of younger forest and the opportunity to hack your way up to the Lake Superior overlook (this spur trail is not groomed). Then Nipisiquit Lake will take what's left of your breath away, and on a sunny afternoon the picnic spot there will tempt you to stay awhile. The second half of the loop continues to climb past wonderful yellow birches. Shortly after you cross the Superior Hiking Trail, you'll head downhill—with enough speed to wish you had goggles.

CAMP TRAILS (6K)

Intermediate and advanced. Watch for signs of wolf as you skirt the hills and lake shores of this rugged terrain on the classic-only trail. It's a long way around Papasay Ridge to get back to Nipisiquit Lake. This may tempt you to ski across the ice on your way back, but do so only with extreme caution, especially near the streams that empty out of or into the lake. Mic Mac Lake is next. If you haven't made your reservation at the cabins on Mic Mac, you will want to do so for next year once you see them. There's a day shelter available to skiers passing through; it's a good stop for a trail lunch. The trail in from the parking lot on Lax Lake Road (Lake County Road 402) is a wide road and can be skated, but is steep enough to keep its intermediate ranking, or even be considered advanced.

TETTEGOUCHE CONNECTOR (6K)

Intermediate. Because of the distance involved and the remoteness, this section should only be skied by experienced and prepared skiers. The first few kilometers are on state park hiking trails and are difficult to groom well, so they might feel more rugged. The Connector follows Smokey Creek's upper reaches in a narrow valley where you'll pass through a gorge with 250-foot walls, eventually linking to the Northwoods Ski Trail. See the Northwoods Ski Trail section for a description of connecting trails and that trailhead.

Flathorn-Gegoka Ski Trails

Isabella, Minnesota

Trailhead access

Six miles west of Isabella on Highway 61, take Highway 1 for 30 miles to Mitiwan Lake Road (Forest Road 177). Then go approximately 0.8 miles to trailhead at Flathorn Lake. Alternately, the Lake Gegoka boat landing may also be used (if plowed); from the boat landing you can ski across the lake to intersection 3.

Total groomed trail: 27.6K

Classic skiing: 27.6K

Trail difficulty

Most of these trails are on old roads, so they're fairly level. On some of the connector routes and around Flathorn Lake, trails get narrower and trickier.

Pass Requirements

• Great Minnesota Ski Pass

Trailhead facilities

Outhouse

Snow conditions

Frequent skier reports at skinnyski.com

What makes it unique

With an abundance of trails providing for a full-day skiing experience, Flathorn-Gegoka is an ideal getaway for guests staying nearby. Trails wind through a beautiful white pine forest, a result of humans and nature working together here—selective forest cutting has allowed these pines to grow especially large.

Information

Superior National Forest, fs.usda.gov

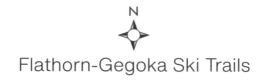

Flathorn-Gegoka Ski Trails

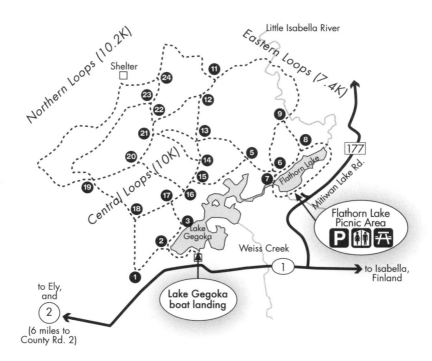

EASTERN LOOPS (7.4K) — INTERSECTIONS 5-13

Intermediate. Entering the trail system from the public access parking, you first ski around Flathorn Lake on challenging trails. Two crossings of the Little Isabella River are especially pretty. Between intersections 9 and 11, the narrow winding trail joins an old road and becomes straighter and flatter all the way to intersection 13. The trail from 5 to 6 and from 6 to 9 is rated most difficult and has steep, curvy hills.

CENTRAL LOOPS (10K) — INTERSECTIONS 1-3, 12-22

Easiest. These loops offer tremendous variety and are situated among the big pines lining old forest roads. East-west connector routes provide lovely skiing with more challenging routes through black spruce bogs and cedar swamps.

NORTHERN LOOPS (10.2K) — INTERSECTIONS 11, 19-24

Intermediate to most difficult. Move out of the white pine and into the realm of red pine trees. These northern loops are all narrow and winding, and may be the last of the system to be groomed. Spruce bogs complete the coniferous diversity. A shelter west of intersection 24 is a good lunch destination if you're on a long outing.

NORTH SHORE SNOW BELTS: GO, SNOW, GO!

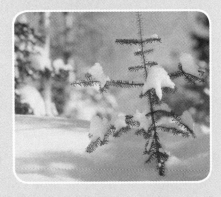

Want huge amounts of fresh, fluffy snow? Then hope for a southeast wind. Although it's rare, a southeast wind draws moisture from open Lake Superior waters. When that moist air reaches land, the cold of the land mass and the height of the shoreline hills draw out the moisture—and it snows like crazy, especially along the ridgeline and inland toward Isabella, Minnesota. So-called "lake-effect snow" can dump up to five feet of snow here, as it did in 1994 in the Silver Bay-Finland area. ❄

North Shore Mountains

Have you ever headed out on your skis and had such a good time you didn't want to stop? Here, you won't have to. Over 200 kilometers of interconnected trails await, linking Tofte nearly to Grand Marais, well up the North Shore. These well-maintained trails weave in and out of the Sawtooth Mountains, and there are tasteful lodges and B&Bs for relaxing along the way. From Carlton Peak to the Cascade River, trails are typically groomed 10 to 15 feet wide by Pisten-Bully groomers. Serious adventurers can head out on the 25K Picnic Loop, families can cruise the Cascade River State Park trails, and skiers seeking slightly wilder experiences can enjoy Bally Creek. There is a trail system here for everyone—don't stop 'til you get to the espresso!

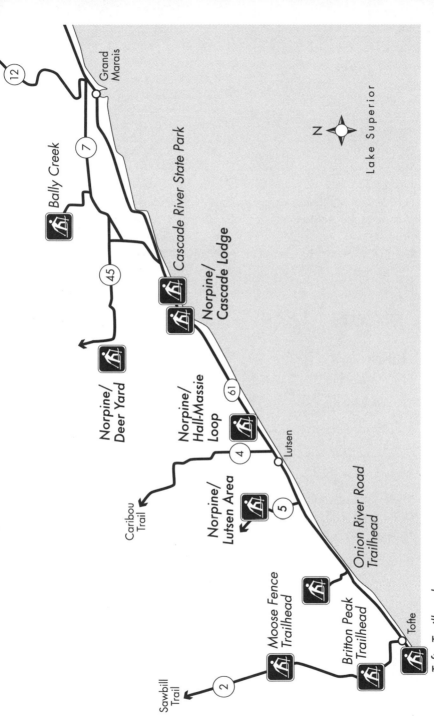

Sugarbush Trail System

Tofte, Minnesota

Trailhead access
(1) Tofte Trailhead: Across from Bluefin Bay Resort on Highway 61, take the Tofte Homestead Road for 0.2 miles. **(2) Britton Peak Trailhead:** From Tofte, take the Sawbill Trail (County Road 2) for 2.7 miles north to Britton Peak trailhead on right, with a large parking area at trailhead. **(3) Moose Fence Trailhead:** From Tofte, take the Sawbill Trail for 7.5 miles north to a small, signed parking lot on the right, directly off road. **(4) Onion River Road Trailhead:** From Highway 61, take Onion River Road (Forest Road 336) for 2.1 miles to a large parking area on left, where the plowed road ends.

Total groomed trail: 65K
Classic skiing: 65K   Skate skiing: 65K

Trail difficulty
Beginning skiers might head for the Onion River Road or Moose Fence trailheads, while intermediate skiers will find their fill at Britton Peak trailhead. All trails are two-way, so please watch for oncoming traffic, especially on steep or curvy sections.

Pass requirements
• Great Minnesota Ski Pass

Trailhead facilities
Outhouses at Britton Peak and Onion River Road trailheads; none at Moose Fence Trailhead. Warming cabin at Onion River Road trailhead.

Snow conditions
sugarbushtrail.org

What makes it unique
Excellent and diverse trails with easy trailhead access and proximity to resorts make this area a popular destination for ski vacations.

Information
Sugarbush Trail Association, sugarbushtrail.org

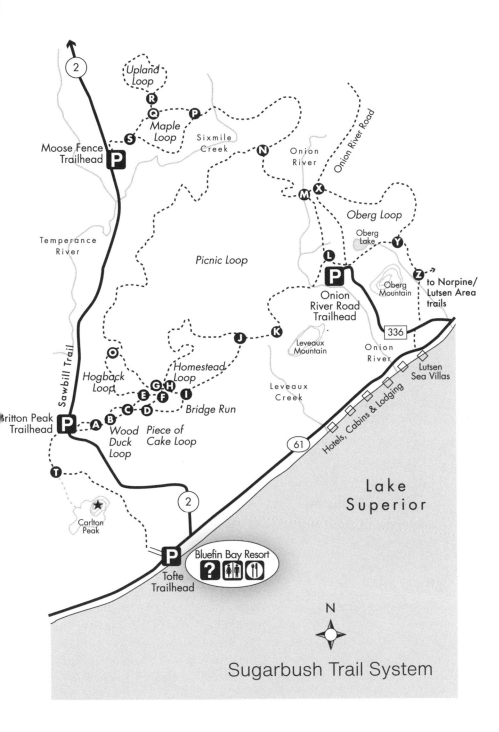

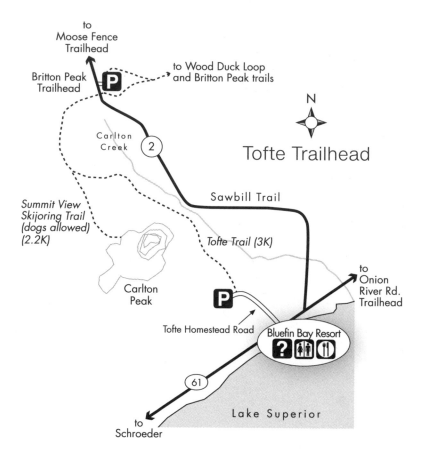

to
Moose Fence
Trailhead

to Wood Duck Loop
and Britton Peak trails

Britton Peak
Trailhead

N

Carlton
Creek ②

Tofte Trailhead

Sawbill Trail

Summit View
Skijoring Trail
(dogs allowed)
(2.2K)

Tofte Trail (3K)

Carlton
Peak

to
Onion
River Rd.
Trailhead

Tofte Homestead Road

Bluefin Bay Resort

61

Lake Superior

to
Schroeder

(1) Tofte Trailhead

*These trails are useful for Tofte resort guests and for skiers with energetic
dogs, including skijorers.*

TOFTE TRAIL (3K)

Intermediate. This trail is best used for so-called "norpine" skiing. Get
someone to drive you to the Britton Peak trailhead, then ski downhill
back to the lake and the Bluefin Bay Resort trailhead. This is a fun run
through a mostly birch forest. Be sure to look off to your right in some of
the open areas for a dramatic view of Carlton Peak and the quarry on its
southeast face.

SUMMIT VIEW (2.2K)

Intermediate/dogs allowed. Follow this summertime road up to the shoulder of Carlton Peak. The trail initially takes you through mostly open country before leading you to the base of the peak. From here you could change to snowshoes and hop on the Superior Hiking Trail to the summit.

SUPERIOR STORM WATCHING

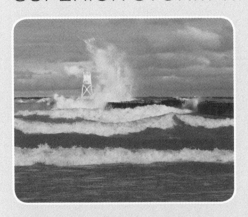

Winter storms on Lake Superior provide one of our more humbling experiences. In a major storm, the lake is so powerful and the gusts are so strong that you feel like dust (or snowflakes) in the wind.

To best experience a roaring northeaster, find a promontory that faces "up" the shore, i.e. northeast. Wear more clothes than normal—the wind chill could easily be many degrees below zero, and you'll want to stay out in the blast for at least ten minutes. Stand in a secure area just close enough to the breaking waves that you can smell the water but not be doused by it, since shifting winds and waves can knock you off your feet.

For great storm watching, try:

- **Duluth's Lakewalk and Canal Park area** near the aerial lift bridge and ship canal piers.
- **Stoney Point.**
- Agate Beach and the picnic area at **Gooseberry Falls State Park.**
- **Shovel Point** at Tettegouche State Park (the 20-minute trail walk from parking lot to Shovel Point will warm you up).
- The **Bluefin Grille in Tofte**, where you can sip coffee and watch the breakers from inside for a slightly more sedate experience.
- Highway 61 parking area at **Cascade River State Park.**
- Artist's Point and East Bay Beach in **Grand Marais.**

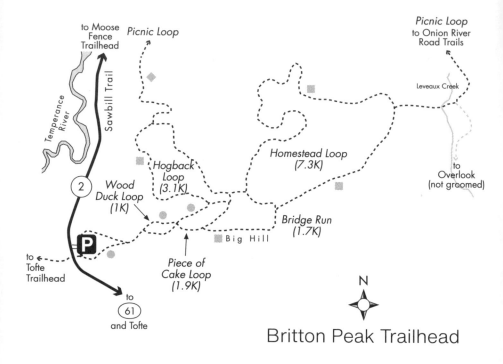

Britton Peak Trailhead

(2) Britton Peak Trailhead

The most popular trailhead on the North Shore, with good reason: there's something here for everyone. Beginners can ski on the first three short loops. Increasingly difficult trails lay beyond, culminating with the majestic Homestead and Hogback Loops.

INNER LOOPS (WOOD DUCK & PIECE OF CAKE LOOPS) (2.9K)

Easiest. Entering the magnificent Sugarbush trails, these first loops are great for warm-ups or for introducing novices to the basics. Aggressive skiers will speed through these loops, but it's worth taking a few minutes to enjoy the views of Carlton Peak through the maples. Wood Duck Loop is named for a small pond it passes with a wood duck nesting box. True beginners should stay on the south part of the first loop to avoid a steep curve right before the trial nears the parking lot.

HOGBACK LOOP (3.1K)

More difficult. If you like a challenge, take the long climb up from the Piece of Cake Loop onto Hogback Ridge. This trail is two-way, but it's better skied clockwise. You'll leave the crowds behind and enjoy some challenging hills. There's one last climb after the junction with the Picnic Loop, then a long, gradual downhill to the end of the loop.

BRIDGE RUN LOOP (1.7K)

More difficult. Here's an introduction to intermediate skiing, with a fast but straight downhill to kick off the loop. The herringbone climb back up to the Piece of Cake Loop is challenging—but you will have more fun continuing around the Homestead Loop for a longer outing.

HOMESTEAD LOOP (7.3K)

More difficult. This makes a great half-day outing. As a counter-clockwise loop it saves the best for last: a 4.5K run through the maples with no stops or intersections, just great views of the Sawtooth mountains both up and down the shore, and two or three fun, short downhills to finish. There are lunch spots all along the loop. Starting and ending at the Britton Peak trailhead, this makes for about a 12K ski.

PICNIC LOOP (25K TOTAL)

Most difficult. This is a classic North Shore ski adventure. The Picnic Loop is an annual ritual for many, a chance to immerse yourself in the woods for a day while experiencing remote country on challenging trails. From the Britton Peak trailhead, it's at least 25K around, depending on which way you take the Homestead Loop. From the Onion River Road trailhead it's about 23K. The Picnic Loop incorporates parts of the Hogback and Homestead loops, the Sixmile Crossing Trail, and adds its own remote 9.2K section of trail. The downhill run after the junction with Sixmile Crossing Trail is an exciting set of switchbacks.

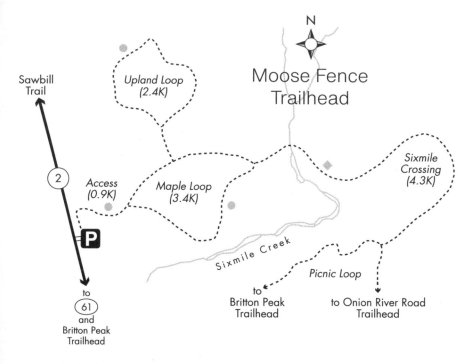

(3) Moose Fence Trailhead

Get away from the crowds, yet enjoy quality grooming and deeper snow. Bring your dog, harness, and leash—this is a popular area for skijoring, dog walking, and romping in the snow.

MAPLE LOOP (4.3K)

More difficult/dogs allowed. A 0.9K access trail takes you from the trailhead up and over a small ridge to the beginning of this loop. The hill down to the start of the loop is the biggest on the whole route. As the name implies, there is primarily maple forest here, but there are also open glades. Take the loop counterclockwise; the south side is a little hillier than the north, and you will climb about 150 feet, though none of it is steep.

UPLAND LOOP (2.4K)

Easiest/dogs allowed. This is what is known as a "lollipop loop." The "stick" of the lollipop is the 0.4K two-way trail at the beginning. And the "candy" part of the lollipop really is sweet: almost 2K of level skiing on top of an easy ridge. Chances are, you'll want to ski this loop twice before heading back. Wildlife signs are common, including moose and a variety of birds.

SIXMILE CROSSING (4.3K)

Most difficult. This section of trail connects Moose Fence with the Picnic Loop and the main Sugarbush region. With a car shuttle, you can enjoy one-way "norpine" skiing from the Moose Fence Trailhead down to the Onion River/Oberg Mountain trailhead. Notice the pure boreal spruce forest in the Sixmile Creek valley: cold air sinks from the maple ridges and keeps out the "riffraff"—trees that can't survive temperatures below -40°F.

WHAT IS A MOOSE FENCE?

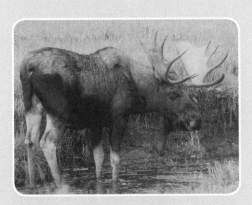

The Moose Fence trailhead is named after a tall fence built here in the 1970s to protect a research plantation of white pine from browsing moose, who love to eat these trees. The fence is gone, but the moose are still here.

The author reports that his closest encounter ever with a moose was here, on the Upland Loop. The adult moose came out of the woods and walked right along the trail. The moose came so near, he could have touched the animal with his ski pole. ❄

Onion River Road
Trailhead

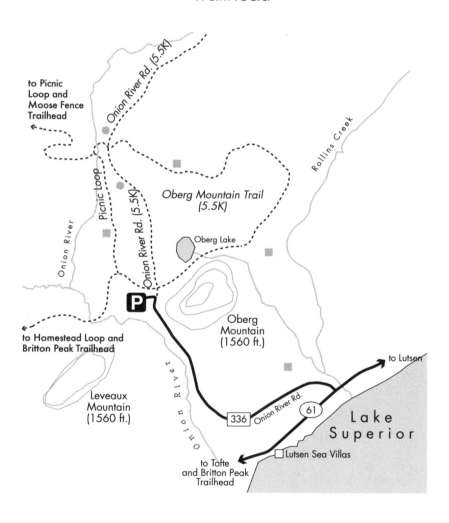

to Picnic
Loop and
Moose Fence
Trailhead

Onion River Rd. (5.5K)

Picnic Loop

Onion River Rd. (5.5K)

Rollins Creek

*Oberg Mountain Trail
(5.5K)*

Onion River

Oberg Lake

P

to Homestead Loop and
Britton Peak Trailhead

Oberg
Mountain
(1560 ft.)

to Lutsen

Leveaux
Mountain
(1560 ft.)

Onion River

336   Onion River Rd.   61

Lake
Superior

Lutsen Sea Villas

to Tofte
and Britton Peak
Trailhead

(4) Onion River Road Trailhead

Between the open views and the rolling trails, skiing this region of trails feels like skiing in the mountains. The cozy, historic cabin at the trailhead was brought down from the top of the Sawbill Trail. You can start a fire in the wood stove, enjoy your lunch or hot cocoa here, then head back out on the ski trails.

HOMESTEAD LOOP (7.3K)

More difficult. From the Onion River Road trailhead, this is a challenging 15K outing and makes a great half-day outing. As a counter-clockwise loop it saves the best for last: a 4.5K run through the maples with no stops or intersections, just great views of the Sawtooth mountains both up and down the shore, and two or three fun, short downhills to the finish. There are lunch spots all along the loop. See Britton Peak Trailhead map for more information.

OBERG MOUNTAIN TRAIL (5.5K)

More difficult. This is a classic climb up into maple forest. Going counter-clockwise, you start with a long climb, then you'll be rewarded with a relatively long level stretch through the thick maples before a quick descent back to the Onion River Road trail. You can return to the trailhead on either the Onion River Road or on a section of the Picnic Loop for an 8.7K total loop.

SUGARBUSH TRAIL ASSOCIATION

Join the Sugarbush Trail Association and help maintain, preserve, and enhance this extensive trail system. As a 501(c)(3) organization, all donations are tax exempt. If you love these fabulously-groomed trails as much as we do, you'll want to contribute to this great cause.

The Association holds meetings in the Tofte area and coordinates beloved events like a candlelit ski & snowshoe evening and the summertime Tofte Trek trail run.

Visit **sugarbushtrail.org** for information and to donate. ❄

ONION RIVER ROAD (5.5K)

Easiest. The trail is groomed nearly wide enough for side-by-side skate skiing. Skiers will enjoy snow here earlier and later than on other trail sections, with skiing some years even into May. During poor snow seasons, this is the best and sometimes only groomed ski trail on the North Shore. One popular option here is to ski up the Onion River Road 2K to Junction X, then turn left for a quick steep run down to Junction M. Turn left again and return through the spruce and meadows to Junction L and the Onion River Road trailhead. Except for the quick downhill run from X to M, this is an easy and very pleasant 4.2K loop.

LODGING IN COOK COUNTY

There are many lodging opportunities in the Lutsen-Tofte area of Highway 61. Learn about resorts, attractions, and events, view maps and a photo gallery, and find complete recreation information on biking, canoeing/kayaking, dogsled rides, fishing, golfing, hiking, horseback riding, and sightseeing at **visitcookcounty.com**.

SPECTACULAR NORTH SHORE MAPLE FORESTS

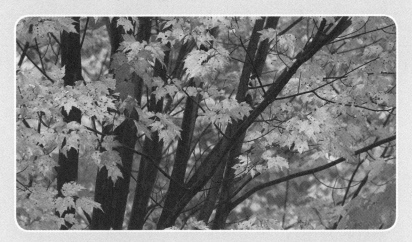

The sugar maples and yellow birches that cover the ridges of the Sugarbush trails are trees of the northern hardwood forest. Given its latitude, the North Shore should be too far north for this sort of hardwood forest. Yet, as any fall color hiker has noticed, sugar maples and yellow birches dominate the Sugarbush landscape.

Anywhere the temperature drops below -45°F, sugar maples and yellow birches cannot survive. The North Shore "should" be a boreal forest of spruce, paper birch, and pine, except for one important factor—the warming influence of Lake Superior. On the ridgelines where sugar maples grow, the warm lake keeps the temperature from dropping to that -45°F killing point, even on the coldest of nights.

In the valleys of the North Shore highlands, the forest is more as it should be for this latitude—with spruce and paper birch species dominating. That's because valleys are frost pockets where the cold air sinking off the ridgeline accumulates and, cut off from the warmth of the lake, reduces the temperature to ranges inhospitable to the yellow birch and sugar maple. So the yellow birch and sugar maple trees live up high; spruce and paper birch trees live down low.

Broadly speaking, the ridges resemble a forest from Central Minnesota (the south) while the valleys resemble a forest in Northern Ontario (the north). The combination of these habitats on the North Shore is nothing less than spectacular. ❄

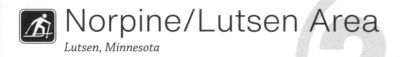

Norpine/Lutsen Area
Lutsen, Minnesota

Trailhead access
There are two trailhead options: **(1)** For the western end, take Ski Hill Road (County Road 5) 1.2 miles inland from Highway 61 to a trailhead on the right side of the road, with limited parking for skiers. The address here is 328 Ski Hill Road. **(2)** For the eastern end, take the Caribou Trail (County Road 4) 1.4 miles inland from Highway 61 and turn left on Homestead Road. Parking is on the right side of the road.

Total groomed trail: 5K
Classic skiing: 5K   Skate skiing: 5K

Trail difficulty
It's hard to get lost on this simple in-and-out trail. It's ranked as "easiest," though there are some climbs and steeper hills at the western end. In low-snow years, the trail has tricky little dips which are more pronounced when snow is low, and the tracks might disappear completely underneath the heavy cedar trees, where snow is shallow or nonexistant.

Pass requirements
• Great Minnesota Ski Pass

Trailhead facilities
None

Snow conditions
norpinetrails.org/TrailsReport.html
facebook.com/NorpineTrails

What makes it unique
This quiet gem in the middle of the busy Lutsen Mountains ski area traverses one of the North Shore's diverse Scientific and Natural Areas. Ample wildlife sign make this perfect for the rambling naturalist on skis.

Information
Norpine Trail Association, norpinetrails.org

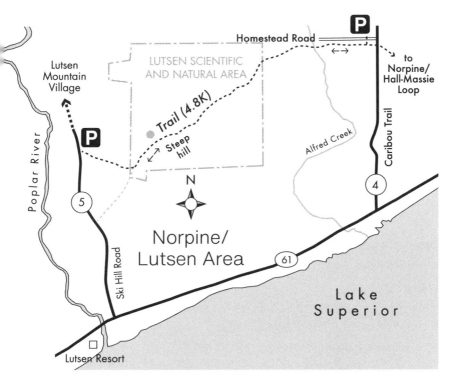

TRAIL (4.8K)

Easiest. According to the Minnesota DNR, the Lutsen Scientific and Natural Area (SNA) is one of the largest blocks of essentially undisturbed old-growth northern hardwood forest in Minnesota. This trail gives you a small sample of the overall SNA. From the Caribou Trail, it's a gradual climb up through yellow birch stands and cedar swamps. When you reach the other end, turn around for a mostly downhill run back. This trail is best in years with ample snow pack because of the many places it travels underneath conifer trees. At the western end there's an intermediate spur down to the Lutsen Recreation rental shop, but there is no parking off of this spur.

Norpine/Hall-Massie Loop

Lutsen, Minnesota

Trailhead access
There are three trailheads: **(1)** Park at Solbakken Resort on Highway 61, milepost 94; **(2)** Drive up Hansen Hjemsted Road from Highway 61 for 0.5 miles to parking lot on the right side of road. **(3)** Take County Road 41 (Hall Road) from Highway 61 for 0.4 miles up to small parking lot on left.

Total groomed trail: 19K
Classic skiing: 19K   Skate skiing: 19K

Trail difficulty
Some of these trails are the flattest you'll find in the area. Others provide long climbs and delicious downhills.

Pass requirements
• Great Minnesota Ski Pass

Trailhead facilities
None. Solbakken Resort has limited public facilities, including a small gift shop.

Snow conditions
norpinetrails.org/TrailsReport.html, facebook.com/NorpineTrails

What makes it unique
The history of homesteading on the North Shore comes alive in these loops named after original settlers. Abraham and Phoebe Massie immigrated from Quebec and worked at a Cascade River logging camp. The Hall family homesteaded in Lutsen in the 1890s off of today's Hall Road, and they are still around.

Information
Norpine Trail Association, norpinetrails.org

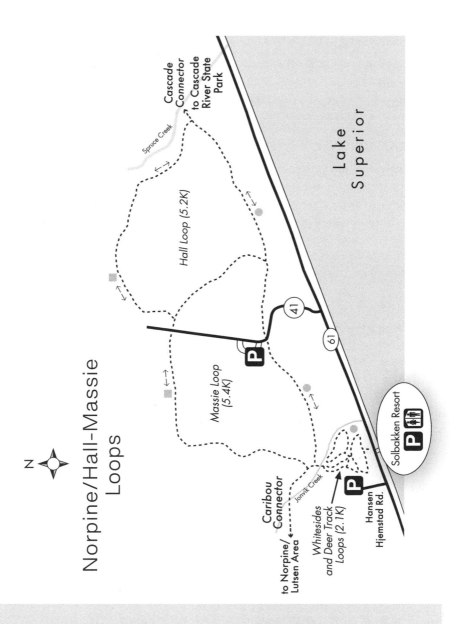

Norpine/Hall-Massie Loops

- N
- Lake Superior
- to Cascade River State Park
- Cascade Connector
- Spruce Creek
- Hall Loop (5.2K)
- 41
- 61
- Massie Loop (5.4K)
- Caribou Connector
- to Norpine/Lutsen Area
- Jonvik Creek
- Whitesides and Deer Track Loops (2.1K)
- Hansen Hjemstad Rd.
- Solbakken Resort

NORDIC + ALPINE = NORPINE

The Norpine Trail Association is a local nonprofit organization that maintains the ski trails found at four trailheads between Lutsen and Grand Marais. "Norpine" is a combination of "Nordic" and "alpine," and refers to the fun downhill trails found in this system. ❄

WHITESIDES/DEER TRACK LOOPS (2.1K)

Easiest and more difficult/classic and skating. The first of these two short loops is the 0.8K Deer Track Loop, named for the deer which frequent the plentiful cedar trees here. This is a flat trail for beginners. Whitesides Loop is a little hillier as it runs along Jonvik Creek.

CARIBOU TRAIL CONNECTOR (1.8K)

More difficult/classic and skating. This is a multi-use trail, where skiers and dogs share the trail with fat bikers. From the Solbakken trailhead, it provides access to Norpine/Lutsen Area trails. It's a 300-foot climb to the Caribou Trail crossing; snow conditions might be less than optimal due to multi-use functionality and lower elevation by the shore. Try it as a in-and-out trail from Solbakken, with a long climb and a challenging descent.

MASSIE LOOP (5.4K)

More difficult. After climbing through an open area and passing the abandoned Massie homestead, enjoy a magical run through a thick grove of cedar.

HALL LOOP (5.2K)

More difficult/classic and skating. Continue from the top of the Massie Loop on the Hall Loop, named after the other family to homestead this area. In contrast with the Massie Loop, this is mostly evergreen trees, including scenic glades of spruce. Like the Massie Loop, the southern part of this loop is open forest, with plenty of openings for wildlife: watch for plentiful deer signs and tracks of the possible wolf that follows.

SOLBAKKEN RESORT

Solbakken Resort offers Lake Superior-adjacent lodging right next to the Hall-Massie Loop trails, and they also offer complimentary ski rental to their guests. Along with Cascade Lodge, this is the heart of North Shore inn-based cross-country skiing, and both resorts connect directly to the Norpine trail system. See **solbakkenon superior.com.**

CASCADE CONNECTOR (to Cascade River State Park) (5.8K)

Easiest. The thru-skier or those who have made shuttle arrangements will enjoy this section connecting Solbakken Resort and the Cascade River State Park trails. Otherwise, it's an in-and-out option.

Norpine/Cascade Lodge

Lutsen, Minnesota

Trailhead access
Cascade Lodge is at Highway 61 milepost 99, ten miles southwest of Grand Marais. Reach the trailhead at the top of the road that leads through the resort, past the cabins.

Total groomed trail: 14.4K
Classic skiing: 14.4K   Skate skiing: 2.5K

Trail difficulty
Medium-wide but twisting trails make for some challenges on this section of the Norpine Trail Association system.

Pass requirements
• Great Minnesota Ski Pass

Trailhead facilities
Full facilities at Cascade Lodge.

Snow conditions
norpinetrails.org/TrailsReport.html

What makes it unique
Cascade Lodge provides true ski-from-your-door lodging, with access from your cabin to over 50K of Pisten-Bully groomed trail in the closely connected Cascade State Park and Norpine/Deer Yard systems.

CASCADE LODGE
Excellent trailside accommodations are found here, including both cabins and lodge rooms, with meals and trail lunches available at the Cascade Lodge restaurant. Lake Superior is a short distance out the door and across the highway. Go to **cascadelodgemn.com** for reservations.

Information
Cascade Lodge, 218-387-1112, cascadelodgemn.com

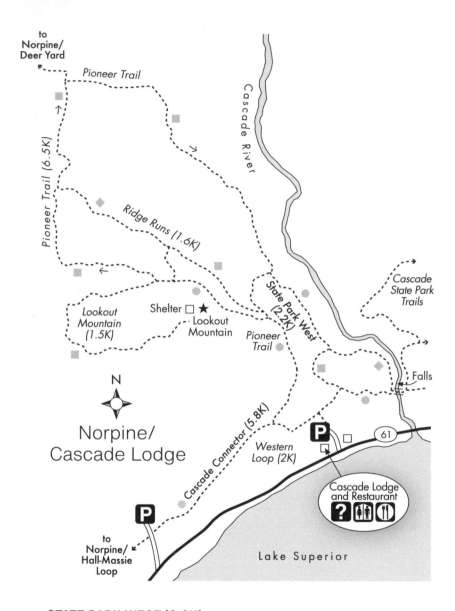

to
Norpine/
Deer Yard

Pioneer Trail

Cascade River

Pioneer Trail (6.5K)

Ridge Runs (1.6K)

Cascade
State Park
Trails

Lookout
Mountain
(1.5K)

Shelter □ ★

Lookout
Mountain

State Park West (2.2K)

Pioneer
Trail

Falls

N

Norpine/
Cascade Lodge

Cascade Connector (5.8K)

Western
Loop (2K)

P

61

P

Cascade Lodge
and Restaurant

to
Norpine/
Hall-Massie
Loop

Lake Superior

STATE PARK WEST (2.2K)

Easiest to advanced/classic only. These are classic, old-fashioned ski trails with tight turns and abrupt, sometimes steep hills. These trails are used extensively by hikers and snowshoers in winter (the Superior Hiking Trail shares the trail). Although the maps show a ski trail connection across the river to Cascade River State Park, you'll have to take your skis off and walk down to the footbridge.

PIONEER TRAIL (6.5K)

Intermediate/classic. This is the primary large loop of the Cascade Lodge system. The first 1.5K are on a wide roadbed, groomed for skating and are rated easiest. After the junction with Lookout Mountain trail, the trail narrows and gets more difficult. Continue on level terrain interspersed with short climbs, past the junction with Upper Ridge Run. You'll reach an elevation of 1,250 feet before descending back into the state park, and to the lodge.

UPPER AND LOWER RIDGE RUNS (1.6K)

Intermediate to advanced/classic only. These are literally runs down a ridge, cutting off from the Pioneer Trail loop. As you approach the last leg of the Upper Ridge Run, have a good snowplow ready as you will be zooming nonstop through a twisting tunnel of balsam fir. There is also a challenging hill midway down the Lower Ridge Run.

LOOKOUT MOUNTAIN (1.5K)

Intermediate/classic only. Take your time on an almost 500-foot climb to the top. The trail narrows and steepens after leaving the Pioneer Trail. After the bulk of the climb, where you will have to herringbone a few times, the trail narrows and then shares space with the Superior Hiking Trail. There is a shelter on top to rest up before the glide down. For a dramatic view of the Cascade River valley, pop your skis off and walk to the scenic overlook about 50 yards past the shelter.

CASCADE CONNECTOR (6K)

Easiest/classic and skating/dog-friendly. This is a multi-use trail also open to fat bikes. It runs wide and level from Cascade Lodge all the way to the Hall-Massie Loop and Solbakken Lodge. This is the best trail option for families and beginners in the Norpine system. There's a small, alternate trailhead about one mile west of Cascade Lodge, off of Highway 61.

Norpine/Deer Yard

Lutsen, Minnesota

Trailhead access
The Deer Yard trailhead is accessed from Cook County Road 7, which runs roughly parallel to Highway 61 from Milepost 101 to the western edge of Grand Marais. Coming from Highway 61 near Cascade River State Park, go 3.2 miles on County Road 7 to the junction of County Road 45 (Pike Lake Road). Turn left here. Go 5.1 miles west on County Road 45. At the intersection of County Road 45 and Murmur Road, continue straight onto Murmur Road (Forest Road #332), 0.7 miles to the trailhead, which is a small parking area on the left side of the road.

Total groomed trail: 18K
Classic skiing: 18K

Trail difficulty
There are no short loops here, so even the intermediate trails become a logistical challenge to prepare for.

Pass requirements
• Great Minnesota Ski Pass
• Donation box at trailhead

Trailhead facilities
None

Snow conditions
norpinetrails.org/TrailsReport.html

What makes it unique
This area is remote and yet very well-maintained, with Norpine Trail Association groomers coming all the way up from Highway 61. The variety of landscape and scenery makes for a great all-day outing.

Information
Norpine Trail Association, norpinetrails.org

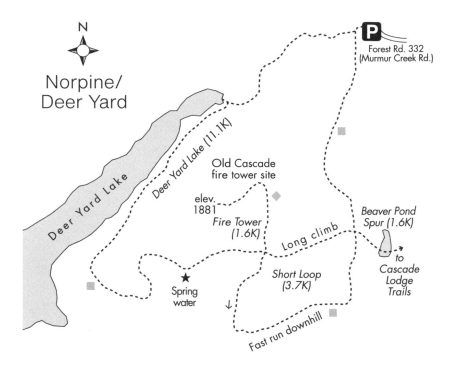

N

Norpine/ Deer Yard

Forest Rd. 332
(Murmur Creek Rd.)

Deer Yard Lake (11.1K)

Deer Yard Lake

Old Cascade
fire tower site

elev.
1881

Fire Tower
(1.6K)

Long climb

Beaver Pond
Spur (1.6K)

to
Cascade
Lodge
Trails

Short Loop
(3.7K)

★ Spring
water

Fast run downhill

DEER YARD LAKE (11.1K)

Intermediate. This is a wonderful half-day trip around a high ridge and along the cedar-lined shore of Deer Yard Lake. The truly ambitious can include this loop as part of a full-day ski up from Cascade River State Park. Traveling counterclockwise, you will experience a variety of forests. Glide down into the old cedars of Deer Yard Lake, and enjoy a break on the lake at its eastern end where a rough trail leads down onto the shore. Stop for spring water in the middle of a North Shore maple and yellow-birch forest. A long hill takes you past the first trail intersection you've encountered in 7K of nonstop skiing. In the last stretch, conifers hold close to the trail.

FIRE TOWER (1.6K)

Advanced. Climb an additional 200 feet to the former site of a fire tower from which there is a good view of Deer Yard Lake. Trail is marked by blue arrows.

SHORT LOOP (3.7K)

More difficult to advanced. Break up your climb on the long loop or, if you are not doing the long loop, take this trail on your way back to the trailhead.

BEAVER POND SPUR (1.6K)

More difficult. A short run along the trail takes you to a wide-open beaver meadow, a nice contrast from the relatively dense forest of the Deer Yard Lake loop. This spur connects Deer Yard with the rest of the Cascade system.

OH, THE BIRDS YOU'LL SEE!

Common birds you are likely to see on a full-day winter outing:
- Black-capped chickadee
- Raven
- Ruffed grouse
- Downy woodpecker
- Red-breasted nuthatch

Birds less frequently seen:
- Pine grosbeak
- Blue jay
- Gray jay
- Bald eagle
- Hairy woodpecker
- Owls, including Barred, Boreal and Saw-whet

Invasive, flocking birds:
- Common redpoll
- Pine siskin
- Bohemian waxwing
- Crossbill ❄

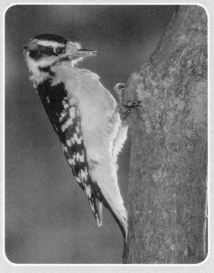

Black and white downy woodpeckers are commonly heard and seen in north shore forests.

Cascade River State Park
Lutsen, Minnesota

Trailhead access
Enter Cascade River State Park at milepost 100 on Highway 61 and take park road to Trail Center.

Total groomed trail: 11.4K
Classic skiing: 11.4K

Trail difficulty
Because of the variety of trails all linked together, this system is best for an intermediate skier who likes a surprise or two. Due to Lake Superior's influence, there may be a big difference in snow depth and snow conditions between the Shoreline Trail and the inland Moose Mountain trails.

Pass requirements
• Great Minnesota Ski Pass
• Minnesota State Park vehicle permit

Trailhead facilities
Restrooms, warming hut

Snow conditions
dnr.state.mn.us/snow_depth/trails.html?facility_id=4112

What makes it unique
This park provides the only North Shore Mountains opportunity for Lake Superior shoreline skiing. Trails are groomed only six feet wide, so you'll feel close to the diverse forest. The quiet little warming shack at the trailhead lets you make a full day of it on these diverse trails.

Information
Cascade River State Park, 218-387-6000
dnr.state.mn.us/parkfinder/index.html

SHORELINE TRAIL (2.8K)

Easiest and more difficult. This is your only opportunity in Cook County and the North Shore Mountains to ski right along the shore of Lake Superior. After dropping down through the (closed) campground and a careful crossing of Highway 61, enjoy a challenging, twisting run a few yards from lake waves or lake ice. Though signed as "easiest," this is actually quite tricky skiing. Snow conditions must be optimal to experience good skiing on this loop.

CEDAR WOODS (6.4K)

Easiest to advanced. This is a great cruise through cedar woods where you'll see numerous signs of deer. One-way trails force you to plan ahead: by skiing clockwise, you can make this a 4K beginner's loop, starting on the river ridge trails. Otherwise, you can climb gradually in a counterclockwise direction, then enjoy either one of two intermediate downhills or a wild advanced downhill (dropping 200 feet in 0.6K). The trails along the edge of the Cascade River Valley offer dramatic views of the valley and Lookout Mountain, set in the pines.

The trail across the Cascade River is quite tricky on skis, and since you don't want to lose control close to the gorge of a rushing river, you'd be best served by taking off your skis and walking here.

MOOSE MOUNTAIN TRAILS (2.2K)

Intermediate to advanced. Depart from the cedar woods and climb another 220 feet to the shelter on top of Moose Mountain. The last section of trail is a real challenge, but the view of Lake Superior is worth it.

BALLY CREEK CONNECTOR (10.4K)

See entry for Wolf Alley in Bally Creek section, p. 122.

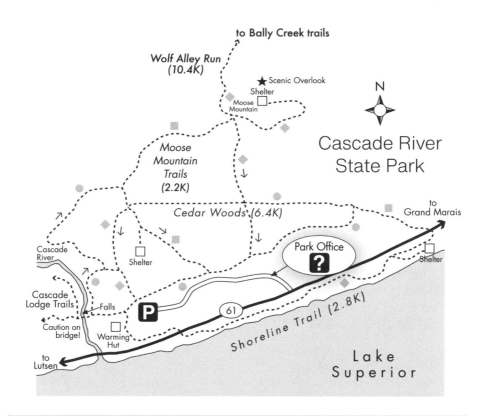

to Bally Creek trails

Wolf Alley Run
(10.4K)

★ Scenic Overlook
Shelter

Moose Mountain

Moose
Mountain
Trails
(2.2K)

Cedar Woods (6.4K)

N

Cascade River State Park

to Grand Marais

Cascade River

Shelter

Park Office
?

Shelter

Cascade Lodge Trails

Falls

P

61

Caution on bridge!

Warming Hut

to Lutsen

Shoreline Trail (2.8K)

Lake
Superior

DEER ARE TOUGH...
AND TOUGH ON TREES

The most obvious wildlife signs you will see in winter are often those of the white-tailed deer. Deer develop and maintain a network of trails through their favorite winter habitat—cedar forests. Deer have four stomachs, allowing them to browse on everything from grass to tree bark, each stomach progressively turning rough plant material into essential nutrients. Because of their voracious browsing to survive the long, cold Minnesota winters, deer are tough on North Shore forests. ❄

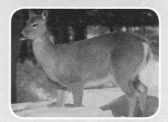

Bally Creek
Grand Marais, Minnesota

Trailhead access
From Highway 61, take Cook County Road 7 about 4 miles to County Road 48, which joins Forest Road 158. Take Forest Road 158 for 2 miles to parking lot on left. This trailhead is shared with a spur of the Superior Hiking Trail.

Total groomed trail: 30.4K
Classic skiing: 30.4K   Skate skiing: 2K

Trail difficulty
Most of these trails are narrower and winding "traditional" ski trails. Although generally level, the trails require some maneuvering. Skinny racing skis are not ideal at Bally Creek.

Pass requirements
• Great Minnesota Ski Pass

Trailhead facilities
None. Cabin rental and lodging information at Bear Track Outfittng.

Snow conditions
Check skinnyski.com trail reports for skier updates

What makes it unique
Rustic cabins allow overnight experiences. Located high up in the North Shore ridges, the Bally Creek trails preserve a traditional skiing atmosphere. As you drive uphill from Highway 61, the snow gets deeper, the forest darker, the road narrower. The trails are over 1,000 feet higher in elevation than Lake Superior, and it feels like a different world here.

Information
US Forest Service trails. Info at Grand Marais ranger station or online at fs.usda.gov/recarea/superior/recarea/?recid=62819

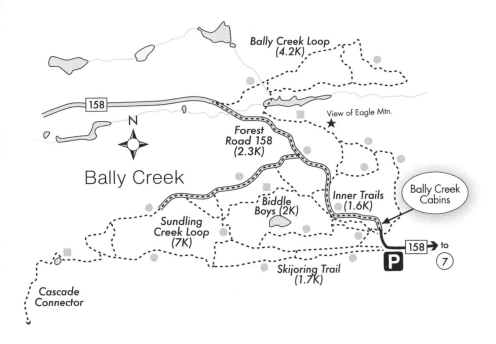

SUNDLING CREEK LOOP (7K)

Easy/classic only. Sundling Creek is a tributary of the Cascade River. The loop starts right at the trailhead parking lot and follows the perimeter of the trail system all the way around to the forest road. The first kilometer, through dense forest, follows an old logging railroad. After this flat and straight stretch, you'll pass a rusty old car. From here the trail gets narrower and a little hillier, including a short but tricky run down to the junction with the Skijoring Trail. After a grove of gorgeous towering aspen and spruce, the trail enters the "Moose Area." This was a clear-cut area but has filled in, so you're not likely to see any sign of moose now. There's a cut-off signed "Moose Yard" trail that shortens the loop. Stay left here and continue past a lovely little pond ringed by cedars. You'll skirt a large area that was logged around 2020. Watch for the "Cascade Connector" trail, aka Wolf Alley, heading off to the left. The loop begins to curve back to the east and enters "The Pines," a large stand of red pine trees. Soon you're on a wide, unplowed forest road. Three separate, narrower trails break off to the right and connect with the Biddle Boys trails. You climb to about 1,650 feet in elevation and gain a wide view over the Sundling Creek valley before descending again to the forest road. It's about 1.5K on the forest road back to the parking lot.

SKIJORING TRAIL (1.7K)

Easy/classic only. Dog-friendly. This trail also leaves right from the trailhead parking lot and parallels the Sundling Creek loop trail. Take the two trails together for an easy 3.7K loop—easy except for the brief connecting trail at the western end.

> # BALLY CREEK CABINS
>
> These wood-heated, rustic cabins are located right within the Bally Creek trail system. Pets are welcome; a separate trail is available for skijoring. Book through AirBNB.

INNER TRAILS (1.6K)

Easy/classic only. Short, winding, classic trails starting from the private cabin trailhead include Rabbit Run, Oscar's Trail, and Wildlife Pond Trail. All are great for a slow warm-up or for wildlife observation.

BIDDLE BOYS TRAILS (2K)

Moderate/classic only. This trail rolls up and down and is generally skier-tracked, without machine grooming. Junctions connect with the Sundling Creek loop. Recommend using wider skis designed for off-trail use.

WOLF ALLEY/CASCADE CONNECTOR (10K)

Moderate/classic only. Find a friend or an innkeeper to deliver you to the Bally Creek trailhead, ski through the system, and enjoy the nearly 1,000-foot drop over 14K or more of trail. The connector takes you through moose and wolf country with beautiful views of Lake Superior.

FOREST ROAD 158 (2.3K)

Easy/classic and skating. This is the continuation of the same road you came in on, unplowed. As a wide and flat Forest Service road, it's perfect for skate skiing. It's also tracked for classic skiing, so bring your first-timers here and ski alongside them.

EAGLE MOUNTAIN OVERLOOK (1.2K)

Moderate/classic only. This is the first of two loops that connect with

Forest Road 158. Taken clockwise, you'll first ski about 1.8K up Forest Road 158 to the signed junction on the right. This is a tricky trail, with steep, narrow hills. Climb to an elevation of 1,700 feet, easily some of the highest terrain in the whole North Shore ski trail system. There is a distant view of Eagle Mountain, the highest point in Minnesota (it's the peak on the right).

BALLY CREEK LOOP (4.2K)

Easy/classic only. This is the second of two loops off of Forest Road 158. The trail winds through deep, impenetrable boreal forest. It's mostly level with a couple of short, steep hills. One section of spruce forest is signed as the "Moose Rub" trail, and you can imagine a large moose barely making it through the trees here.

If you take the loop counter clockwise, you cross scenic Bally Creek Pond right away. This is a short, ungroomed stretch that might not be passable early in the season. If so, start and end the loop another 200 yards further down Forest Road 158. .

THE PRESENCE OF WOLVES

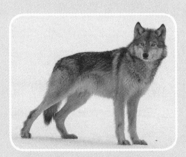

As you glide along a ski trail, an odd, primordial feeling might shake you particularly alert to your surroundings. You might notice a tuft of brown or white fur, floating loose in the breeze. Maybe you see an odd combination of critter tracks in the snow, like deer and raven tracks. Perhaps there is a grove of cedar trees ahead. A tingle runs up your spine; the hair on the back of your neck bristles. Soon not just a tuft of brown fur is visible but a clump of hide, too. The groomed ski tracks are trampled underneath a chaos of animal markings—maybe there are comb-marks from the wing tips of ravens, and wolf scat still fresh, brown, and moist. Just off the ski trail in that grove of cedars, you see what's left of a white-tailed deer laying in the snow. The ravens are in the trees, squawking. Are the wolves crouching somewhere, silently watching and waiting as you gingerly ski around their recent prey?

This not-uncommon trail discovery marks the end of one life and the continuance of many others—life and death in the North Shore forest. We are so lucky to ski amidst the wildness of wolves. ❄

Gunflint Trail

Take a short drive up and away from the North Shore to arrive at heaven. This is the wild Boundary Waters, complete with remote lakes, rugged land...and cross-country ski trails. The resorts of the Gunflint Trail have assembled a pure skiing experience, from their dueling Pisten-Bully groomers to their saunas, heated trail shelters, and wax rooms. Whether you are gliding around Pincushion Mountain, circling Central Gunflint lakes, or climbing Upper Gunflint ridges, you will be immersed in skiing and skiing only. Finish your tour with a ski on the Banadad Trail, staying in a yurt along the way, and you will have enjoyed a complete Gunflint Trail experience.

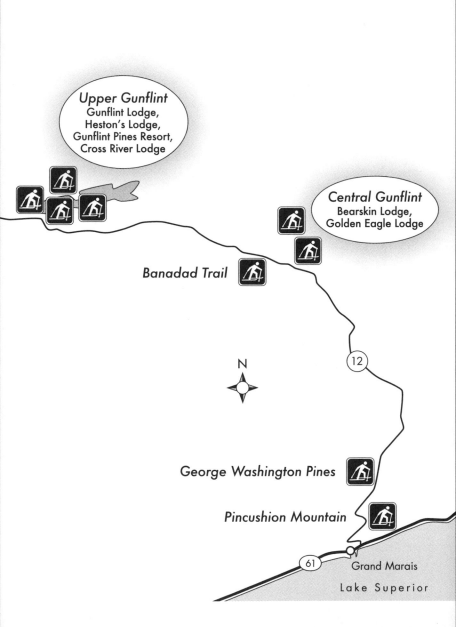

Pincushion Mountain

Grand Marais, Minnesota

Trailhead access
Take Gunflint Trail 1.7 miles north from Highway 61 in Grand Marais and enter the Pincushion trailhead road on right.

Total groomed trail: 23K
Classic skiing: 23K   Skate skiing: 23K

Trail difficulty
Consistent grooming and wide trails make this system accessible for all levels, although the longer loops and steeper hills are better for more advanced skiers.

Pass requirements
• Great Minnesota Ski Pass
• Recommended donation of $5/person/day to support the North Superior Ski and Run Club, which administers this trail system. A yellow donation box is located on the main entrance sign, just below the warming chalet.

Trailhead facilities
Outhouse, warming chalet at public trailhead

Snow conditions
pincushiontrails.org
facebook.com/Pincushion-Mountain-Trails

What makes it unique
These are some of the only trails on the shore designed by skiers specifically for cross-country skiing, and it shows. The trails have a real community feel, from the tourists sharing the fabulous parking lot view to the sign that lists the Grand Marais businesses that support the North Superior Ski and Run Club.

Information
North Superior Ski and Run Club, pincushiontrails.org

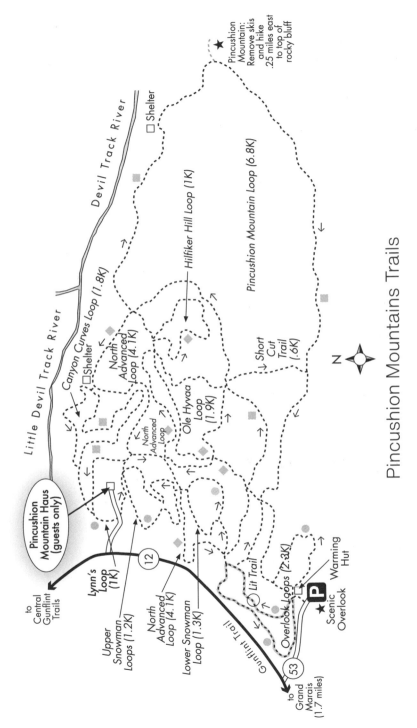

Pincushion Mountains Trails

Pincushion Mountain: Remove skis and hike .25 miles east to top of rocky bluff

Devil Track River

☐ Shelter

Little Devil Track River

Hilfiker Hill Loop (1K)

Pincushion Mountain Loop (6.8K)

Canyon Curves Loop (1.8K)

☐ Shelter

North Advanced Loop (4.1K)

N

Short Cut Trail (.6K)

Ole Hyvaa Loop (1.9K)

North Advanced Loop

Pincushion Mountain Haus (guests only)

Lynn's Loop (1K)

to Central Gunflint Trails

12

Upper Snowman Loops (1.2K)

North Advanced Loop (4.1K)

Lower Snowman Loop (1.3K)

Lit Trail

Overlook Loops (2.3K)

Warming Hut

Gunflint Trail

P

★ Scenic Overlook

53

to Grand Marais (1.7 miles)

GUNFLINT TRAIL: **Pincushion Mountain 127**

OVERLOOK LOOPS (2.3K)

Easier/partly lighted. These two loops start and end at the public trailhead and are named for their location near this overlook, rather than for any view from the trails themselves. The West Overlook Loop (1.3K) is lighted at night; a steady climb starts it off. The dog-friendly East Overlook Loop, at 1K, is separated from the rest of the traffic but is a little hillier than the west loop, making it less suited for real beginners.

PINCUSHION MOUNTAIN LOOP (6.8K)

Intermediate. Follow the signs through the first four intersections as you head out on this loop. Although rated intermediate, this trail offers relatively easy skiing and provides a perfect morning or afternoon outing through a mature birch forest. Stretch out the day: snack at the shelter overlooking the Devil Track River valley, take off your skis to walk 0.25 miles to the top of Pincushion Mountain, and discover a wide view of Lake Superior from the summit.

NORTH ADVANCED LOOP (4.1K)

Advanced. This loop is carved out of the hilly central section of this trail system; once again, the well-done signage allows you to skip reading maps and simply follow the arrows. Ski this loop a couple of times and watch for the transition into and out of a nearly pure birch forest from a mixed aspen, spruce, and fir forest.

LOWER AND UPPER SNOWMAN (2.5K)

Easier. Carved into the existing trail network in 2004, these three loops are stacked on top of each other like, well, a snowman. Although surrounded by advanced trails, these are easy, open loops.

LYNN'S LOOP (1K)

Easier. This trail is perfect for guests of Pincushion Mountain Haus to try out their skills before heading out on the advanced trails.

CANYON CURVES LOOP (1.8K)

Intermediate. This trail lives up to its name right away as you descend from Lynn's Loop down a curvy trail. The trail loops and turns through birch and fir before a final run along the rim of the Little Devil Track River. Take a second loop around before you grunt back up the hill.

OLE HYVAA AND HILFIKER HILL LOOPS (2.9K)

Advanced. These are rolling trails in the tradition of adventurous Nordic skiing, as seen in their names. The 1.9K Ole Hyvaa Loop is loosely translated from the Finnish for "Oh my God!" The 1K Hilfiker Hill Loop is named after Dr. Hilfiker, an early ski enthusiast who lived near the trails in the early 1970s.

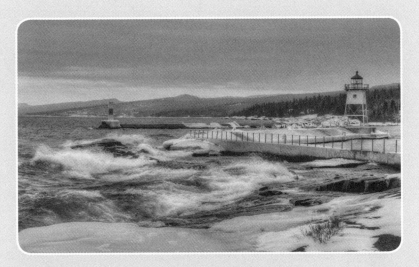

IT'S NEVER A BAD DAY IN GRAND MARAIS

It's raining in February, the result of an unusual warm spell. Or it's ten below zero and the wind is howling. You could go skiing, but something says you're not that crazy. Instead, head into town and enjoy some North Shore culture.

Cruise the aisles of Joynes Ben Franklin Department Store for woolen wear, toys for the kids, or unique shoes. Check out art of the north at Sivertson Gallery or the Johnson Heritage Post. Sip a micro-brew at the Gunflint Tavern. Enjoy a Blizzard at Dairy Queen. A day in Grand Marais without skiing is not so bad, after all. ❁

George Washington Pines

Grand Marais, Minnesota

Trailhead access
Take Gunflint Trail 7 miles north from Highway 61 in Grand Marais to parking lot on left.

Total trail: 3.5K
Classic skiing: 3.5K

Groomed once a week, this trail is open to all uses including snowshoeing and dog walking.

Trail difficulty
You'll enjoy easy skiing on level trails here, and you might find dog and human footprints in your ski tracks.

Pass requirements
• None

Trailhead facilities
None

Snow conditions
Check skinnyski.com trail reports for skier updates

What makes it unique
This gentle little loop provides a quiet alternative to the large trail systems typical of the Gunflint region. This pine plantation was planted in 1932 by Boy Scouts from Grand Marais to reforest an area hard hit by logging and fires.

Information
Superior National Forest, Gunflint Ranger District, 218-387-1750
fs.usda.gov

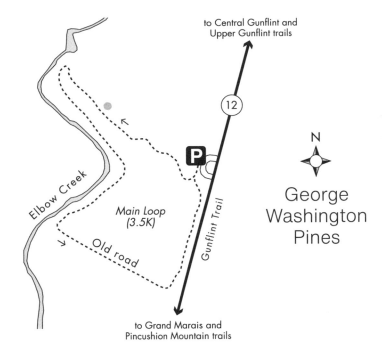

to Central Gunflint and
Upper Gunflint trails

12

N

George
Washington
Pines

Elbow Creek

Main Loop
(3.5K)

Gunflint Trail

Old road

to Grand Marais and
Pincushion Mountain trails

MAIN LOOP (3.5K)

Easier. Although groomed only occasionally, this simple loop is used often enough by both local skiers and respectful snowshoers that you can generally count on a decent trail. The counterclockwise loop starts and ends in the pine plantation for which it is named, but along the way there is a wide variety of forest types, as well as mellow little Elbow Creek.

PEACEFUL PINES

This forest was planted on George Washington's 200th birthday, in 1932. He might have been proud to see how skiers, snowshoers, and walkers all peacefully coexist on this trail.

Groomed ski trails typically do not fair well with snowshoers or dogs present, but everyone loves to get out in these snowy woods. Follow simple rules posted at the trailhead—skiers head counterclockwise on the trail, snowshoers keep clear of the ski tracks, dog owners leash your dog and remove waste—and everyone can share and enjoy this National Forest trail. ❀

Central Gunflint

Grand Marais, Minnesota

Trailhead access

Take the Gunflint Trail north from Grand Marais to either: **(1) Bearskin Lodge:** Drive 26 miles on the Gunflint Trail, take right at Bearskin Lodge sign, continue short distance to Lodge office; or **(2) Golden Eagle Lodge:** Drive 28 miles on the Gunflint Trail, take right on Clearwater Road, continue for 3.5 miles to Lodge office.

Total groomed trail: 55K

Classic skiing: 55K   Skate skiing: 34K   Lighted trail: 2.1K

Trail difficulty

You'll find a bit of everything here, from flat and wide beginner trails to steep and twisty expert terrain.

Pass requirements

• This trail system is privately owned and free for guests of Bearskin Lodge and Golden Eagle Lodge. For others, daily pass $18 ($12 after 1pm); 3-day pass $36; and season pass $100. Children 13 and under receive reduced rates. Available at trailheads.

Trailhead facilities

Full facilities at both trailheads, including snacks and ski rental. Trail maps provided when buying tickets at trailhead offices.

Snow conditions:

facebook.com/GoldenEagleLodge, golden-eagle.com (trail webcam) bearskintrailreports.com

What makes it unique

Two lodges cooperate here to maintain an excellent and vast network of trails ideally suited for a family cross-country ski vacation. Half of the trails are considered intermediate.

Information

Golden Eagle Lodge, golden-eagle.com; Bearskin Lodge, bearskin.com

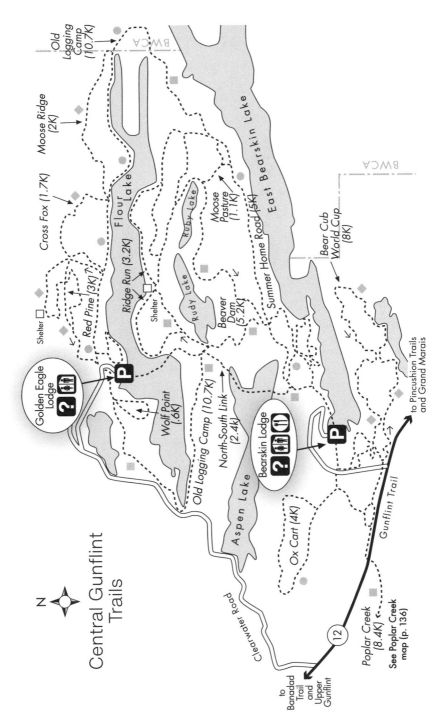

Central Gunflint Trails

N

Old Logging Camp (10.7K)

BWCA

Moose Ridge (2K)

Cross Fox (1.7K)

Flour Lake

Red Pine (3K)

Shelter

Ridge Run (3.2K)

Shelter

Ruby Lake

Rudy Lake

Moose Pasture (1.1K)

Beaver Dam (5.2K)

East Bearskin Lake

Summer Home Road (5K)

BWCA

Bear Cub World Cup (8K)

Golden Eagle Lodge

?

P

Wolf Point (.6K)

Old Logging Camp (10.7K)

North-South Link (2.4K)

Aspen Lake

Bearskin Lodge

?

P

Ox Cart (4K)

to Pincushion Trails and Grand Marais

Gunflint Trail

Clearwater Road

12

Poplar Creek (8.4K)

See Poplar Creek map (p. 136)

to Banadad Trail and Upper Gunflint

Bearskin Lodge Area Trails

SUMMER HOME ROAD/CAMPGROUND (5K)

Easier/classic and skating/partially lighted. This is the central corridor for Bearskin Lodge area trails, and because it is built on roads, it can be groomed more aggressively than other sections. When conditions are marginal everywhere else in northern Minnesota, this may be the only good skiing you will find. It is wide and mostly level, good for families and beginners. The 1999 blow down is quite obvious on the eastern end of this trail. A combination of parts of the Beaver Dam Trail, Summer Home Road and North-South Link form a 1.5K loop lighted at night by a string of Christmas lights.

OX CART TRAIL (4K)

Easier to Intermediate/classic only. This "lollipop loop" is mostly easy, intimate skiing. Since it's groomed only for classic striding, classic skiers can enjoy the quiet woods at their own pace. After crossing a beaver pond, the trail climbs gently into pine woods. Take the whole loop back to the lodge and you've skied 5.2K.

BEAR CUB WORLD CUP (8K)

Advanced/classic and skating.
If you want a wild ride and are ready to push yourself, this is the trail to test your abilities. Think Lycra and wild aerodynamic sunglasses—the trail was designed specifically for challenging skate skiing, including steep uphills and "screaming" downhills.

CENTRAL GUNFLINT LODGING

Bearskin Lodge and Golden Eagle Lodge both offer excellent accommodations for skiers and direct access to the trails they jointly manage. Cozy lodging and true ski-from-the-door convenience is found at both.

Bearskin Lodge
218-388-2292
bearskin.com

Golden Eagle Lodge
218-388-2203
golden-eagle.com

POPLAR CREEK (8.4K)

Easier to Intermediate/classic only. This loop (see map p. 136) makes for a round trip of 10.2K from the junction with the Oxcart Trail. The loop takes you away from the main network of trails, across the Gunflint Trail into a quiet country of small lakes, bogs, and meandering streams. A shelter halfway around makes a nice break on a day-long outing. The northern part of this section is also the beginning of the Banadad Trail (see p. 138).

NORTH-SOUTH LINK (2.4K)

Advanced/classic and skating. Although half of this trail is on the flat surface of lakes, it earns an advanced rating due to steep hills and the potential hazards of lake skiing. Stay on the groomed trails and, if in doubt about lake ice conditions, ask at one of the lodges before heading out.

Golden Eagle Lodge Area Trails

OLD LOGGING CAMP (10.7K)

Easiest to advanced/classic and skating. This is the main part of a 13–14K loop around Flour Lake. East of Golden Eagle Lodge the trail follows an old logging railroad leading to the site of a historic logging camp, complete with "timber jays." After a brief and hilly passage over the boundary of the BWCA, the trail disappears into the Bearskin-area trail network. The trail reemerges on the west end of Rudy Lake for a wild ride on top of glacial eskers around the end of Flour Lake. You can cut this loop in half with the North-South Link.

WOLF POINT (0.6K)

Intermediate/classic only/lighted. This is Golden Eagle Lodge's night skiing loop illuminated by electric lights. Hills that are fun by day are thrilling at night.

NORTH FLOUR LOOPS (6.7K)

Advanced/classic and skating. Three side trails roll off an easy section of the Old Logging Camp trail. Each side trail climbs through blowdown forest to ridges with views both south over the lakes and north into Canada. The Red Pine loops total 3K, lead through blow down and a

Central Gunflint Trails: Poplar Creek

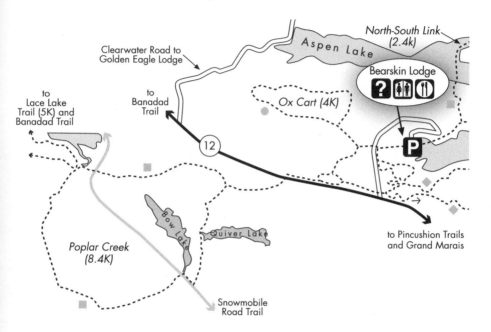

young red pine forest, and have a shelter on top with a view of West Bearskin Lake. The Cross Fox Trail has 1.7K of up and down. Finally, Moose Ridge offers a steep climb to Canadian views and a roller coaster ride back down to Old Logging Camp trail.

MOOSE PASTURE (1.1K)

Easier/classic and skating. Open woods here are the result of forest management and the 1999 blowdown storm, providing good winter habitat for moose. You may be visited by gray jays when you stop for a snack; bring some extra peanuts, just in case.

RIDGE RUN TRAIL (6K)

Intermediate to advanced/classic only. This trail runs along the ridge overlooking Flour Lake. Watch for sharp turns and great views. The overlooks on Flour Lake are dramatic and might make you exclaim, "It looks just like the Boundary Waters!"

BEAVER DAM TRAIL (5.2K)

Easier to intermediate/classic only. Loop clockwise around Rudy and Ruby Lakes on this varied trail. There are some wild downhills along the southern part of the loop. You can really see the varied effects of the blowdown storm here. There is a shelter halfway around, overlooking Flour Lake.

THE 4TH OF JULY BLOWDOWN, 1999

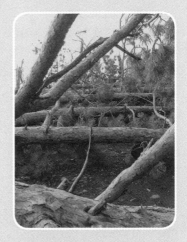

In 20 minutes, powerful forces claimed centuries of old-growth forest and set the stage for decades of forest recovery. Straight-line winds of up to 100 miles per hour flattened almost 500,000 acres of forest from Ely to the Gunflint Trail. What had been a deep, intimate forest before the storm became a tangled web of fallen tree trunks, eventually turning into open, logged areas.

The visual impact on Gunflint ski trails was dramatic. Over half of the trails here lead through blowdown areas. While the cross-country skiing remains great as ever here, the visual evidence of the big blow will last for decades. ❀

Banadad Trail

Grand Marais, Minnesota

Trailhead access

The main access is at the Poplar Creek Guesthouse B&B, two miles off the Gunflint Trail on the Lima Grade (Forest Road 315) and the Little Ollie Road. At the western end, there is parking at Rib Lake Road, 0.25 miles southeast of Loon Lake Public Landing.

Total groomed trail: 36K

Classic skiing: 36K

Trail difficulty

The Banadad is generally a level and easy trail, but because it heads through remote wilderness areas, is best for experienced skiers only.

Pass requirements

• Great Minnesota Ski Pass
• BWCA Wilderness day-use permit (available at wilderness boundary or through outfitters).

Trailhead facilities

Bed and breakfast or yurt accommodations.

Snow conditions

banadad.org

What makes it unique

This is the region's premiere wilderness trail experience, providing a wonderful combination of groomed trails and deep wilderness, plus unusual accommodations in yurts—complete with Mongolian dinners.

Information

Banadad Trail Association, banadad.org

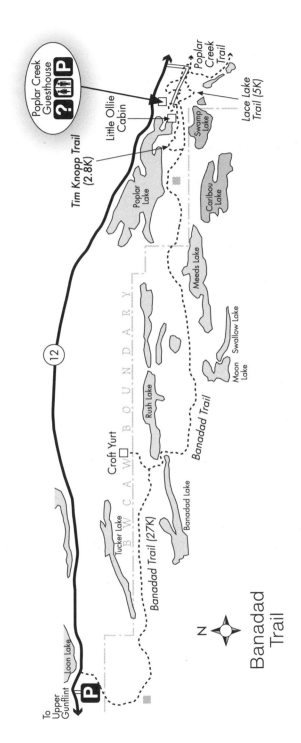

Poplar Creek
Guesthouse

? 🅿

Little Ollie
Cabin

Tim Knopp Trail
(2.8K)

Poplar
Creek
Trail

Lace Lake
Trail (5K)

Swamp
Lake

Poplar
Lake

Caribou
Lake

Meeds Lake

Swallow Lake

Moon
Lake

12

B W C A W   B O U N D A R Y

Banadad Trail

Rush Lake

Croft Yurt

Banadad Lake

Banadad Trail (27K)

Tucker Lake

Loon Lake

To
Upper
Gunflint

🅿

N

Banadad
Trail

Here it is, the ultimate combination of groomed trail and wilderness skiing. The Banadad Trail is 27K of nearly pure wilderness experience. Most skiers will want or need to break up the trip by staying overnight in a yurt or a cabin operated by Boundary Country Trekking. They say that "Banadad" means "lost" in Anishinaabe, but don't worry: the trail is well marked and well groomed.

The trail runs entirely across land, not across frozen lakes, so slush is not a concern. For a few miles in the middle, the trail follows the Laurentian Divide, which separates the Lake Superior watershed from the Hudson Bay watershed. In the western end, look for beaver ponds, while throughout the trail you will find open spruce bogs and dense forest. Cliffs parallel the trail at times.

The trail was created in the early 1980s out of logging roads left over from before 1978, the year logging was banned in the BWCA. The old roadbed provides a smooth skiing surface, and remnants of old logging camps give you history to ponder. Before the major national long-distance ski races became dominated by skaters, the Banadad was often used as training for races such as the Birkebeiner. But no one should race through this wonderful country anymore. Take your time and enjoy a backcountry classic.

You can arrange the all-important shuttle via the Poplar Creek Guesthouse B&B or with other lodges.

BANADAD TRAIL LODGING

Complete your Banadad Trail experience by staying overnight in a yurt or trailside cabin. Spend your first night at the eastern end, at Tall Pines Yurt, Little Ollie cabin or in the Poplar Creek Guesthouse. Then head west on the trail to the Croft yurt, where your bags await you. The last day, your car will be waiting for you at the western end of the trail.

For more information, visit Boundary Country Trekking. boundarycountry.com.

TIM KNOPP TRAIL (2.8K)

Easier. This trail is well suited for guests staying at the Poplar Creek Guesthouse B&B or Little Ollie Cabin. The Tim Knopp Trail was named for a University of Minnesota professor and skier who was vital to the renaissance of skiing.

LACE LAKE (5K)

Easier to intermediate. The casual visitor to Banadad country may ski this loop as part of a long day's outing from Bearskin Lodge off the Poplar Creek Trail, but to get the full experience, visit Ted and Barb Young at Poplar Creek Guesthouse B&B. This loop takes you right up to the edge of the BWCA and along scenic Poplar Creek.

TALL PINES (1.7K)

Easier. Ski to (or from) the Tall Pines Yurt, past big white pines.

THE HAM LAKE FIRE, SPRING 2007

In these woods, the only constant is change. Severe drought conditions plus potential fuel from the 1999 blowdown storm made for dangerous fire conditions in May of 2007.

A human-caused fire started near a campsite at Ham Lake, right by the Ham Lake ski trail. After burning north past Seagull Lake, the fire burned near the Magnetic Rock Trail, crossed into Canada, and looped around the north shore of Gunflint Lake. Then, a tongue of the fire ran back along the eastern side of Gunflint Lake and Loon Lake, crossed the Gunflint Trail, and burned near Rush Lake and the middle of the Banadad Trail. Over 74,000 acres were burned in the U.S. and Canada.

The upper Gunflint Trail was evacuated and the fire destroyed over 100 buildings. The dramatic story is grippingly recounted in the book *Gunflint Burning: Fire in the Boundary Waters,* by Cary Griffith.

Fortunately, no lives were lost and the lodges reopened. Skiing on the Gunflint Trail remains excellent, and when you ski on these trails, you'll be witnessing ecological history. ❀

Upper Gunflint

Grand Marais, Minnesota

Trailhead access
Take the Gunflint Trail to the Upper Gunflint lodges (see map). Once you have a pass, you can start at Loon Lake Boat Access or the Scenic Overlook on the Gunflint Trail, in addition to the lodges.

Total groomed trail: 66.5K
Classic skiing: 66.5K   Skate skiing: 17.4K

Trail difficulty
There is not much trail here for a true beginning skier, but there is a lot of challenging terrain for the more experienced skier.

Pass requirements
• Passes available at all resorts ($15/day adults; $8/day kids). Price includes trail map.

Trailhead facilities
Full facilities at resort trailheads. Rental available at Gunflint Lodge. All skiers should check in and buy their passes at the resorts.

Snow conditions:
gunflint-trail.com

What makes it unique
Like the Central Gunflint system, the Upper Gunflint system is an amazing skiing resource, with ski-from-your-door convenience and an incredible variety of terrain. These trails are better for experienced skiers, since there are few beginner trails near the lodges.

Information
See lodge listings on p. 146.

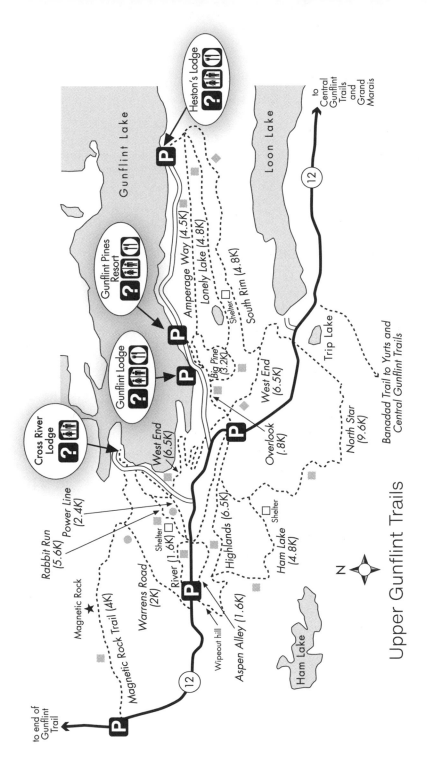

Upper Gunflint Trails

Cross River Lodge

Gunflint Lodge

Gunflint Pines Resort

Heston's Lodge

Gunflint Lake

Loon Lake

Trip Lake

Ham Lake

Rabbit Run (5.6K)

Power Line (2.4K)

Magnetic Rock

Magnetic Rock Trail (4K)

Warrens Road (2K)

River (1.6K)

Shelter

Wipeout hill

Aspen Alley (1.6K)

Highlands (6.5K)

Shelter

Ham Lake (4.8K)

West End (6.5K)

West End (6.5K)

Overlook (.8K)

North Star (9.6K)

Big Pine (3.2K)

Amperage Way (4.5K)

Lonely Lake (4.8K)

South Rim (4.8K)

Shelter

Banadad Trail to Yurts and Central Gunflint Trails

to Central Gunflint Trails and Grand Marais

to end of Gunflint Trail

N

12

Northwest trails, accessed from Cross River Lodge or Warrens Road parking area

POWER LINE (2.4K)

Easiest/classic only. This double-tracked trail provides access to the trails for guests of Cross River Lodge and vacation homes along County Road 46 (unfortunately, from Cross River Lodge you'll need to use the road to cross the Gunflint Lake bay) and makes for an accessible loop through Aspen Alley, Warrens Road and the Cut Across Trail.

WARRENS ROAD (2K)/CUT ACROSS TRAIL (1.6K)

Easier to intermediate/classic only. Warrens Road is an easy and fast double-tracked trail that runs from a gravel pit to a three-way intersection with the Magnetic Rock Trail. The Cut Across Trail is rated more difficult, but the cautious beginner should have no problem and enjoy these gradual hills.

MAGNETIC ROCK (4K)

Intermediate to advanced/classic only. From the intersection with the Cut Across Trail, this remote trail leads past a small pond, a fire burn, and a 60-foot high glacial erratic that will make your compass needle swing. There is a parking lot on the Gunflint Trail at the far western end of this trail, but the trail may not be groomed all the way through. Ask locally about this trail; the Ham Lake Fire of 2007 burned right through here.

ASPEN ALLEY/RIVER TRAIL (3.2K)

Easier to intermediate/classic only. These two trails combine on either side of the Gunflint Trail for a relatively easy, open country loop. You can park off the road at the western end of the trails. The River Trail, on the north side, is better suited for more experienced skiers, running up and down an esker beside scenic Cross River. There are few aspens standing in Aspen Alley, but you get a great view of the hillside where they were all blown down in 1999.

Corridor Trail

WEST END TRAIL (6.5K)

Intermediate to advanced/classic and skating. Think of this trail as a big freeway connecting all destinations. It connects the River Trail on the west with Loon Lake on the east. Along the way, the trail is hilly and challenging with some very steep climbs and descents, dramatic views, and intimate forests. The eastern half was mostly untouched by the blowdown storm.

Gunflint Lodge and Gunflint Pines trails

BIG PINE (3.2K)

Easier to Intermediate/classic only. Climb a steep hill from Gunflint Lodge on a broad trail through blowdown forest, then everything changes into a magic grotto of deep green ringed by steep cliffs. Dramatic scenery and signs of wildlife make this loop a great introduction to Gunflint-style skiing.

LITTLE PINE (2K)

Easier to intermediate/classic only. This is a small loop trail between Gunflint Lodge and Gunflint Pines. It winds through barns and access roads, all in blow-down areas.

RABBIT RUN (5.6K)

Easier to Intermediate/classic and skating. Branching off the West End Trail, this double-tracked trail runs along the bottom of a glacial ridge, past a luxury trailside shelter, then crosses the Gunflint Trail paralleling the Highlands Trail below the 140-foot cliff. The shelter is worth planning your day around: it is set between a cliff and a spruce bog and has propane heat, an indoor picnic table, and even a rack for your skis.

OVERLOOK (0.8K)

Easier to Intermediate/classic and skating. This short, hilly, double-tracked trail is your access to not only the scenic overlook but to all the trails on the south side of the Gunflint Trail. There's no real view at the overlook, but keep climbing on the trail to the Highlands Trail, over

300 feet up from the lodges, and you'll find a huge view through extensive blowdown areas of the lakes below.

SOUTH RIM (4.8K)

Intermediate to advanced/classic only. Stride along the top of a ridge with dramatic views of Gunflint Lake, 400 feet below, and the Canadian hills beyond. You could use the Lonely Lake Trail as part of a round-trip return. Steep hills at both ends keep this section in the advanced category. Not recommended during low-snow conditions.

LONELY LAKE (4.8K)

Easier to Intermediate/classic only. This double-tracked trail runs parallel to the South Rim Trail, but far below, beside pretty cliffs. The climb up at the eastern end from Heston's Lodge is particularly dramatic, with old-growth white pines and pleasant views of Gunflint Lake. A luxury warming hut is located near the west end of the trail.

UPPER GUNFLINT TRAIL LODGING

The lodges on Gunflint Lake all provide excellent accommodations for skiers.

Cross River Lodge
196 N. Gunflint Lake Road,
Grand Marais MN 55604,
218-388-2233.
crossriverlodge.com

Gunflint Lodge
143 S. Gunflint Lake Road,
Grand Marais MN 55604
218-388-2294
gunflint.com

Gunflint Pines Resort
217 S. Gunflint Lake Road
Grand Marais MN 55604
218-388-4454.
gunflintpines.com

Heston's Lodge
579 S. Gunflint Lake Road,
Grand Marais MN 55604
218-388-2243
hestons.com

AMPERAGE WAY (4.5K)

Intermediate/classic and skating. This is the best skating trail in the Upper Gunflint system. It parallels the Lonely Lake trail. Groomed eight-feet wide, it's meant for skaters and skijorers. The trail goes through a thick cedar swamp.

Trails south of the Gunflint Trail

HIGHLANDS TRAIL (6.5K)

Intermediate to advanced/classic and skating. Hills at both ends of this double-tracked trail bracket a high-country run with nice views all along the way. The preferred travel direction is from east to west, allowing you to pause for views as you climb from the scenic overlook on the Gunflint Trail, and providing for the full experience of Wipeout Hill—with an "S" curve and drop of over 120 feet to the Cross River, below.

HAM LAKE TRAIL (4.8K)

Easier to Intermediate/classic only. Take a detour from the Highlands Trail and get into some serious moose country. The gently rolling, double-tracked terrain is well suited for novice skiers, but there are intense climbs to get here, so be forewarned. Most of this trail was untouched by the blowdown storm, and includes beautiful stretches of jack pine. Another luxury warming hut will come in handy for a snack break. Ham Lake itself is down below the trail, but is never actually visible.

NORTH STAR (9.6K)

Intermediate/classic only. Diverse habitats marked this trail even before the blowdown storm, including forestry management areas, wetlands, and dense forests. After a pleasant descent to a crossing of Ham Creek, it's mostly open country. Cross the Gunflint Trail at the eastern end.

Acknowledgements

This book would not have been possible without the tireless work of the hundreds of winter recreation lovers who groom the trails in winter, clear and build them in the summer, and promote their use year-round.

Special thanks to Lisa Angelos of Jay Cooke State Park and Ben Croft of Cloquet Nordic.

In Wisconsin, a tip of the cheesehead to Linda Cadotte for her support of the Superior Municipal Forest, and to Josh McIntyre of the Brule River State Forest.

In Duluth, thanks to the late Kelly Fleissner of the City of Duluth, to John Paulson, and to the Duluth Cross-Country Ski Club (especially Siiri Morse). Each time I talked with Glen Nelson on the Piedmont trail, he shared another bit of great history and passion. At Hartley Park, Gary Larson helped with a thoughtful redesign of the trail system, which turned the damages from a major blowdown storm into a modern trail.

Al Ringer is the long-time steward of the Mother Bear trails and is always helpful with updates.

John Kron and Mark Gordon in Two Harbors are groomers and advocates for the Erkki Harju trails.

At Tettegouche State Park, Gary Hoeft was a constant source of information. But I will never forget Sam Cook and Ann Harrington, who joined Sally and me for a great winter's trek on the Tettegouche Connector so long ago.

Katie Foshay, park manager at Split Rock Lighthouse State Park, provided guidance on the changing status of those lakeshore trails.

Kudos to Andy Fisher and Lura Wilson, who kept the Flathorn-Gegoka experience alive.

In the amazing Tofte area trails, the Sugarbush Trail Association continues to maintain a world-class system. Jeff and Sarah Lynch at Sawtooth Outfitters have responded to my strangest questions and rented the right gear to my big-city nephews during their visit.

Norpine volunteers Timothy B. Nelson and Thom McAleer are keeping the vital links of Lutsen, Cascade, and Deer Yard alive and well, picking up where Bill and Beth Blank and Michael and Maureen O'Phelan left off.

Heading up the Gunflint Trail, Scott Beattie and Bob Nesheim helped me see Pincushion from their inside views. Generations of the Baumann family at Golden Eagle Lodge hosted our family adventures. Lee Kerfoot's Gunflint Lodge was my base for exploring the Upper Gunflint Trails with their North Woods hospitality. Barb and Ted Young from the Banadad Trail spent a lot of time with me and continue offering their great hospitality.

On a personal note, I want to share that my parents, Dick and Ella Slade, introduced me to the Sugarbush Trail System 30 years ago. And our sons literally grew up on most of these trails, from riding in infant backpacks to racing at high school ski meets.

But my beautiful wife and skiing companion, Sally Rauschenfels, is the true genius of this book. It was her vision that created it and her motivation that has seen it through. I would have lost the trail long ago without her.

Andrew Slade
Duluth, Minnesota

About the author

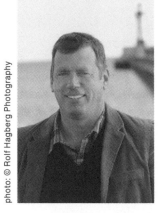

Andrew Slade's parents first set eyes on each other on the North Shore, and his life has centered there since birth—despite growing up in the Twin Cities. As a kid, he caught nets full of smelt at the Cross River, jumped cliffs into the deep pools of an unnamed North Shore river, helped to band woodcock in the open fields of North Shore homesteads, and shut his eyes tight each time the family wagon drove around Silver Cliff (readers, don't worry— today there's a tunnel through the cliff and his eyes stay wide open). With his intrepid father, he had to abandon a mid-1970s assault on Carlton Peak due to a lack of recognizable trails.

As a canoe guide and outdoor educator in Ely, he learned that "sauna" is a three-syllable word (sow-ooh-nah). In his twenties, he bushwhacked by snowshoe much of what is now the Manitou-Caribou section of the Superior Hiking Trail. At age 28, in his "before kids" era, he was the editor and lead author of the first *Guide to the Superior Hiking Trail*.

Slade graduated from the University of Minnesota with a BA in environmental education and from the University of Montana with a MS in environmental studies. His favorite wildflower is *Mertensia paniculata*, the native North Shore bluebell.

Andrew has worked for environmental education, parks and conservation organizations on the North Shore since 1992. Reach him at andrewhslade@gmail.com.

About There and Back Books. We live and play in northern Minnesota—a fabulous landscape filled with wild rivers, deep woods, diverse wildlife, and the greatest Lake. An abundance of great trails, campgrounds, state parks, outfitters, and lodging makes this landscape accessible to nearly everyone. Our guidebooks feature detailed maps, dozens of photographs, and descriptive text to boost your confidence and get you safely "out there"...and back. We'll see you on the trail!

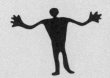

THERE AND BACK BOOKS READ. GO. DISCOVER.

bestnorthshore.com
Your guide to Minnesota's spectacular Lake Superior region

Camping the North Shore

A guide to the best campgrounds in Minnesota's spectacular Lake Superior region SECOND EDITION

By Andrew Slade $16.95

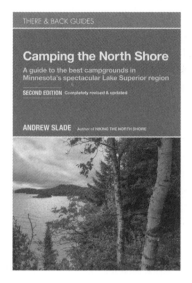

Leave the ordinary behind— camp Minnesota's North Shore

Naturalist and outdoors expert Andrew Slade scouted out nearly two thousand campsites in this spectacular region, seeking unique and beautiful places to camp. *Camping the North Shore* not only guides you to the best of the best, it gives you fun activities and adventures for each location, complete with detailed maps and dozens of photographs. This guidebook will help you enjoy Lake Superior views, catch nice fish, relax in peace and quiet, and find an ideal base camp to boat, hike, or even shop on the North Shore.

For RV and tent campers, seasoned experts, and those new to camping—find your perfect place in the woods.

From Jay Cooke State Park to the Gunflint Trail, from convenient campgrounds in town to wilderness campgrounds on the edge of the BWCA, this guidebook features the 26 "best" North Shore campgrounds and describes 35 more — that's 61 campgrounds in all!

Camping the North Shore not only guides you to the best of the best, it gives you fun activities and adventures for each location, complete with detailed maps and dozens of photographs. **- Beth Gauper, MIDWESTWEEKENDS.com**

Campers will discover a ton of useful information crammed into this 134-page book...with honest, matter-of-fact descriptions. **- Shawn Perich, NORTHERN WILDS MAGAZINE**

Camping the North Shore provides for those who want their up-close-and-personal visit to include their down-time...This is a good guide to help take the guesswork out of a camping trip. **- Monica Isley, LAKE COUNTY NEWS-CHRONICLE**

Hiking the North Shore

50 fabulous day hikes in Minnesota's spectacular Lake Superior region SECOND EDITION

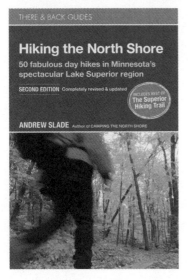

By Andrew Slade, $16.95

Get into Minnesota's most rugged and scenic wild places. Gear up for the best hiking in the Midwest!

Naturalist and North Shore expert Andrew Slade scouted out over 300 miles of trails along inland ridges and Lake Superior shoreline for this indispensable guide. Grab your boots and go!

Those new to Minnesota's North Shore, as well as experienced hikers in Lake Superior country, will find *Hiking the North Shore* the most comprehensive resource around—Andrew hiked every trail, checked out every overlook, and visited every waterfall so you can plan a perfect day's hike. Find recommendations for short and easy hikes that will quickly plunge you into a true North Shore experience, as well as longer, more challenging hikes that will take you to the highest points in Minnesota, unusual geological formations, and old-growth forests. *Hiking the North Shore* will encourage and inspire hikers of all skill levels to get out and explore these beautiful routes. What are you waiting for?

Everything you need is inside this book:

- Details on day hikes ranging from 2 miles to 12 miles.
- Driving directions to trailheads.
- Maps of each hike with time estimates for every hike.
- A full range of hikes—trails perfect for families with young kids, challenges for hard-core adventure seekers, and moderate hikes for everyone else.
- Information on facilities, permit requirements, and helpful websites.
- Suggestions for timing your hike for spring wildflowers, summer berries, or fall colors...with fascinating lore about flora, fauna, geology, and history.
- Tips for planning round-trip and shuttle hikes.
- Recommendations for kicking back after your hike, including nearby restaurants, lodging, camping, and museums.